EXERCISE IDEAS

for

Upper Body Strengthening

edited by
Dr. Irv Rubenstein

VISUAL HEALTH INFORMATION
Tacoma, WA

Cover design by Roxanne Carrington
Publication design and layout by Bethany Maines
Illustrations from the libraries of VHI

10 9 8 7 6 5 4 3 2 1

Printed in the United States of America

Publisher's Cataloging-in-Publication
(Provided by Quality Books, Inc.)

Exercise ideas for upper body strengthening / edited by Irv Rubenstein.
    p. cm.
    ISBN 1-929343-05-1

    1. Exercise.   I. Rubenstein, Irv.

GV508.E948 2005   613.7'1
                         QBI05-200073

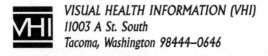

VISUAL HEALTH INFORMATION (VHI)
11003 A St. South
Tacoma, Washington 98444-0646

Book Orders: 1-800-356-0709
All Other Inquiries: 1-253-536-4922

CONTENTS

Introduction 1

Chapter 1: Chest Exercises 1

    Push-ups 2

    Presses 5

    Machines 8

    Isolations (Flies, Raises, Diagonals) 10

    Tubing 13

    Stability Ball 16

    Medicine Ball 18

    Aquatic 20

Chapter 2: Shoulder Exercises 22

    Presses 23

    Anterior Deltoid 26

    Middle Deltoid 29

    Posterior Deltoid 31

Chapter 3: Upper / Middle Back Exercises 34

    Tubing 35

    Dumbbells 39

    Barbells 43

    Machines 44

    Cables 46

Chapter 4: Latisimus Dorsi Exercises 49

    Pulls 50

    Dips 54

    Sweeps 56

    Aquatic 58

Chapter 5: Biceps Exercises 60

Dumbbells 61

Barbells 66

Machines / Cables 68

Tubing 70

Chapter 6: Triceps Exercises 71

Press-ups 72

Dips 73

Dumbbells 75

Barbells 78

Tubing 81

Machines / Cables 83

Chapter 7: Abdominal Exercises 86

Calisthenics 88

Machine / Weights 94

Stability Ball 97

Tubing 100

Medicine Ball 101

Chapter 8: Low Back Exercises 104

Calisthenics 105

Stability Ball 108

Tubing 111

Weights 113

Machines 115

Medicine Ball 117

Chapter 9: Forearm Exercises 121

Flexion 122

Extension 125

Rotation 127

Lateral / Medial Deviation 128

Chapter 10: Rotator Cuff Exercises 129

Internal Rotation 130

External Rotation 134

Diagonals 139

Scaption 141

Periscapulars 142

Stablization / Proprioception 144

Chapter 11: Neck Exercises 147

Extension 148

Flexion 151

Rotation 154

Lateral Flexion 155

Chapter 12: Finger / Hand Exercises 158

Finger / Hand 159

Introduction

The material in this collection of 524 upper body strengthening exercises is designed to meet the needs of medical and fitness professionals who work with the strength needs of patients and clients.

Therapists and trainers often have limited resources – either working with a minimum of gym equipment or in people's homes. Creativity becomes more important under these circumstances. When a client's unique needs or interests confront a therapist or trainer, his/her understanding of biomechanics and anatomy may be challenged in ways that require him or her to search for options. This collection was designed and should be used to find ways to get the same results with a variety of methods.

This collection of upper body exercises will provide the trainer with over 524 exercises for the muscles and joints above the waist, exclusive of the abdominal and spinal structures. The content for this book was derived from the extensive exercise database of Visual Health Information (Tacoma, WA). It is not the purpose or intent of this collection to represent each and every possible exercise option for each part of the body. Nor is it the intent to describe and define when and how to use or not use any one exercise for any particular client's or athlete's needs, especially where a therapeutic consideration is warranted. Rather, it is designed simply as a resource, a reference for medical and fitness professionals who have an in-depth knowledge of exercise prescription principles.

For simplicity, the chapters are laid out in an orderly fashion with an attempt to minimize crossover. For example, a bench press is used for developing four muscle groups: pectoralis major, anterior deltoid, serratus anterior, and the triceps. It will be included in each section related to each muscle group; that is unavoidable.

Finally, as in any book of this nature, a disclaimer is necessary. Thus, anyone using the exercises listed in this book without appropriate training in the field of rehabilitation, exercise science or fitness, or, without the prior consent of a physician or therapeutic professional, may be placing his/her clients or him- or herself at risk for an injury. The exercises are provided as options, not prescriptions, and are therefore to be used in concert with an experienced professional's education and guidelines.

Chapter 1: Chest Exercises

The chest is comprised of one large superficial muscle – the pectoralis major, or pec – and a smaller, less visible muscle – the coracobrachialis, rarely noted even on the bodybuilder. The pec is often considered a two-part muscle, with the upper portion designated as the clavicular head, and the lower portion as the sternal head. Since it inserts on the upper humerus, its main role is to move the shoulder. It flexes and adducts the shoulder and, when the arm is overhead, assists in pulling it back down as an extensor. There are no motions in which it acts in isolation; shoulder muscles and some of the upper arm muscles act in concert with it.

Chest exercises include one or more of the following muscles: Pectoralis Major, Serratus Anterior, Anterior Deltoid, Triceps, Biceps, and Latissimus Dorsi.

Push-Ups – 12 exercises
Presses – 11 exercises
Presses (Machine) – 5 exercises
Isolations (Flies, Raises, Diagonals) – 11 exercises
Tubing – 11 exercises
Stability Ball – 6 exercises
Medicine Ball – 8 exercises
Aquatic – 6 exercises

Wall Shoulder Press-Out

With palms flat on wall, shoulder-width apart, and elbows straight, press shoulders back. Return.

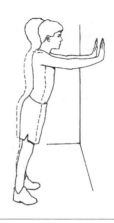

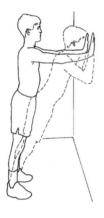

Wall Push-Up

With feet and hands shoulder-width apart, lean into wall, then push away from wall.

Wall Push-Up: Single Arm

Stand away from wall with one hand on wall. Perform a push-up.

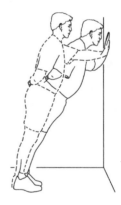

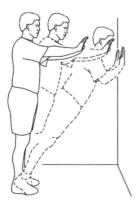

Closed Chain: Wall Push-Off

Stand away from wall. Fall toward wall, absorbing impact with arms. Immediately push back to start.

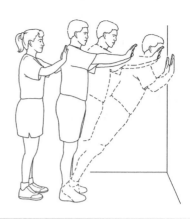

Wall Push-Off: Assisted

Stand away from wall, partner behind. Partner pushes you toward wall. Absorb impact with your arms. Immediately push back. Partner stops you and pushes back toward wall.

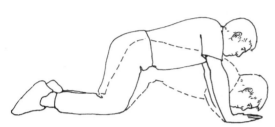

All Fours Push-Up

On all fours with hands shoulder-width apart, bend elbows and perform a push-up. Return to start position.

All Fours Push-Up with Press-Up

On all fours with hands shoulder-width apart, bend elbows and perform push-up. Return and press shoulders up, arching upper back. Return.

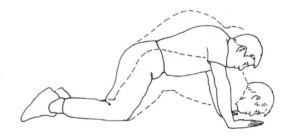

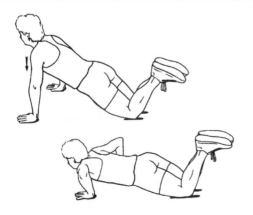

Modified Push-Up

From starting position with knees bent, hands outside shoulder width and body straight, lower body until chest touches floor.

Push-Up Position Press-Up

In push-up position, press shoulders up. Then sag down to start position.

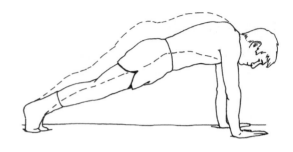

Push-Up

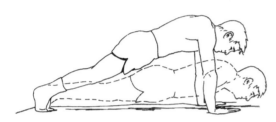

With toes on ground, feet together, hands shoulder-width apart, and chest on floor, push up by straightening arms. Then lower body slowly to start position.

Push-Up with Press-Up

With toes on ground, feet together, hands shoulder-width apart, and chest on floor, push up by straightening arms. Continue by pressing up shoulders and arching upper back. Return to start position with chest to floor.

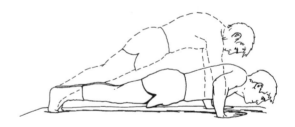

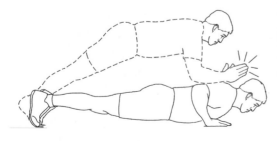

Push-Up: Clap

Start from lowered position of push-up. Forcefully push up out of this position. Clap hands before returning to start.

Bench Press (Dumbbell)

Press to straight arms.

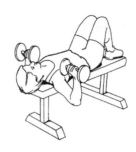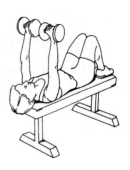

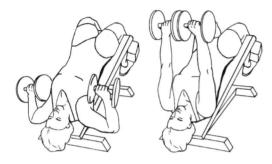

Bench Press: Decline (Dumbbell)

Press to straight arms.

Bench Press: Incline (Dumbbell)

Press to straight arms.

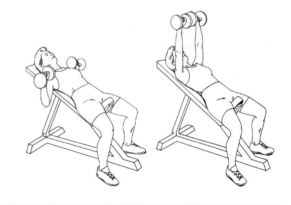

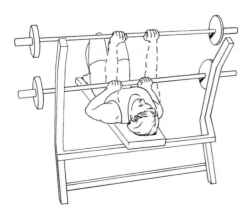

Bench Press: Narrow Grip (Barbell)

Press to straight arms.

Bench Press: Medium Grip (Barbell)

Press to straight arms.

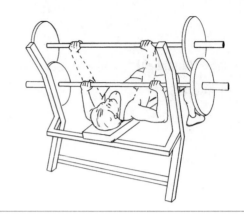

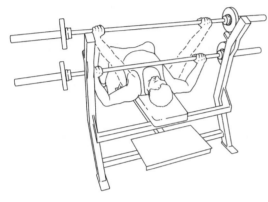

Bench Press: Wide Grip (Barbell)

Press to straight arms.

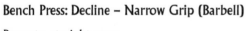

Bench Press: Decline – Narrow Grip (Barbell)

Press to straight arms.

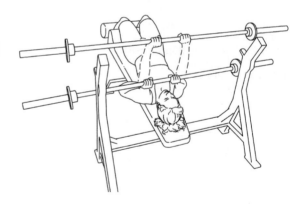

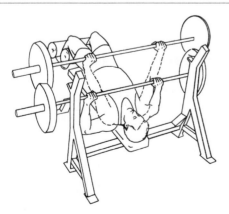

Bench Press: Decline – Medium Grip (Barbell)

Press to straight arms.

Bench Press: Decline – Wide Grip (Barbell)

Press to straight arms.

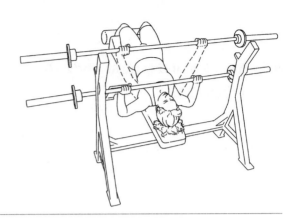

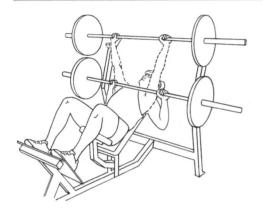

Bench Press: Incline – Medium Grip (Barbell)

Press to straight arms.

Bench Press: Incline – Narrow Grip (Barbell)

Press to straight arms.

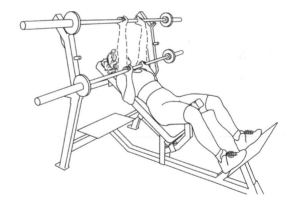

Bench Press: Medium Grip (Smith Machine)

Press to straight arms.

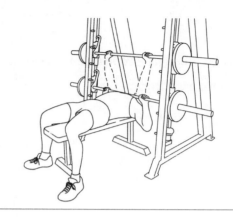

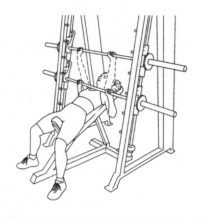

Bench Press: Incline – Medium Grip (Smith Machine)

Press to straight arms.

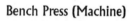

Bench Press (Machine)

Press to straight arms.

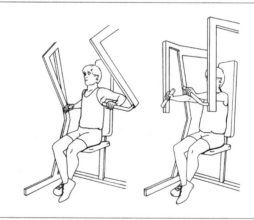

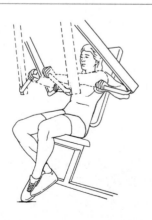

Bench Press: Decline (Machine)

Press to straight arms.

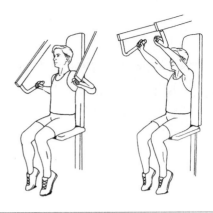

Bench Press: Incline (Machine)

Press to straight arms.

Front Deltoid Raise: Single Arm (Dumbbell)

Knees slightly bent, raise dumbbell over head, keeping elbow locked. Alternate arms.

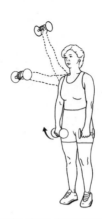

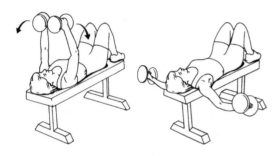

Fly (Dumbbell)

Lower arms until parallel with floor, elbows slightly bent, palms up.

Fly: Decline (Dumbbell)

Elbows slightly bent, lower arms until parallel with floor, palms up.

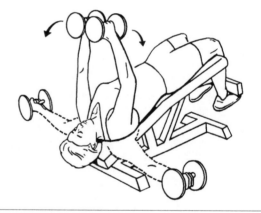

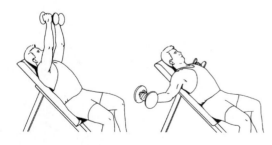

Fly: Incline (Dumbbell)

Elbows slightly bent, lower arms until parallel with floor, palms up.

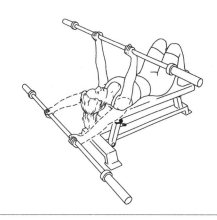

Pull-Over: Straight Arms – Medium Grip (Barbell)

Lower arms until parallel with floor, keeping arms nearly straight.

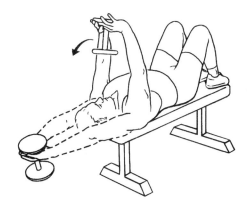

Pull-Over: Straight Arms (Dumbbell)

Lower arms until parallel with floor, keeping arms nearly straight.

Fly: Lying (Cable)

Cross arms over middle chest, keeping elbows slightly bent.

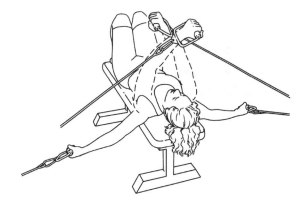

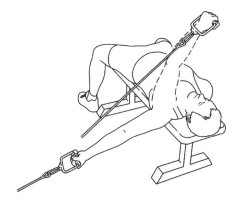

Fly: Lying – Single Arm (Cable)

Cross arm just past midline of body, over middle chest, keeping elbow slightly bent.

Fly: Standing (Cable)

With loose grip, cross arms just past midline of body under lower chest, keeping elbows and knees slightly bent.

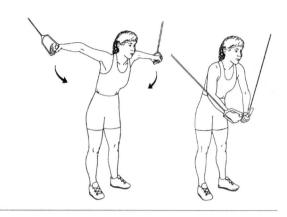

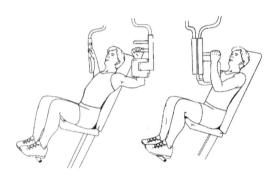

Fly: Decline (Machine)

Bring handles together, keeping elbows bent to 90°.

Fly (Machine)

Bring handles together, keeping elbows slightly bent.

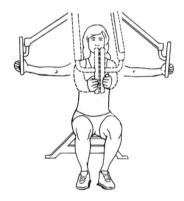

Chest Press

In shoulder width stance with tubing behind back and hands in punch position, press arms straight ahead.

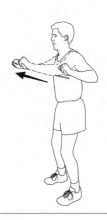

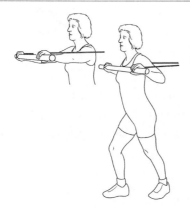

Wall Push-Up: Standing – Resisted

In shoulder width stance, lean to wall, band anchored under hands. Push away.

Chest Press: Incline

In shoulder width stance with tubing behind back and hands in punch position, press arms ahead and up.

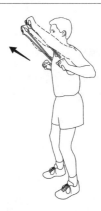

Chest Press

Face away from anchor in stride stance. Grasp bar, palms down. Press arms out.

Push-Up: Modified – Resisted

Tubing looped behind back and anchored around hands, lean forward in kneeling position, arms bent. Push up by straightening arms. Keep knees on floor.

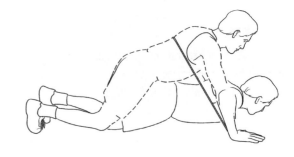

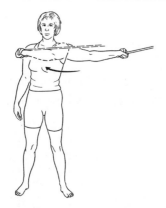

Push-Up: Resisted

Tubing looped behind back and anchored around hands. Push up from floor on toes by straightening arms.

Strengthening: Resisted Flexion

Hold tubing with arm at side. Pull forward and up. Move shoulder through pain-free range of motion.

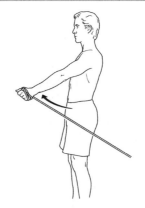

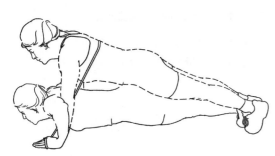

Strengthening:
Resisted Horizontal Adduction

Hold tubing in hand, elbow straight, arm out, parallel to floor. Bend elbow 90° then pull arm across body through pain-free range.

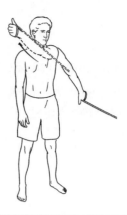

Strengthening: Resisted Diagonal

Hold tubing with arm down and out from side, thumb down. Pull arm across body and over head, rotating arm to thumb up.

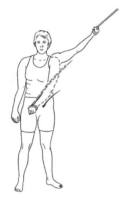

Strengthening:
Resisted Diagonal Extension

Hold tubing with arm above and behind, palm up. Bring arm down across body, rotating to palm down.

Functional Pattern Strengthening: Forehand

Hold tubing with hand behind and out. Pull hand forward while pushing arm out as in tennis forehand.

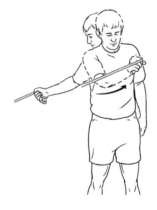

Wall Push-Up: Single Arm (Gymball)

Stand away from wall, one hand supporting a gymball on the wall. Perform a push-up.

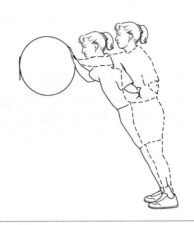

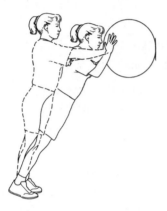

Wall Push-Up: Double Arm (Gymball)

Stand away from wall with both hands supporting a gymball on the wall. Perform a push-up.

Prone Push-Up from Mid-Thigh

Roll forward until ball rests under thighs. Perform push-up. Keep back straight.

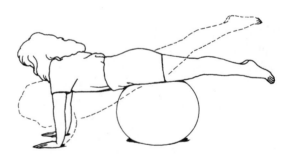

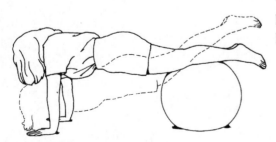

Prone Push-Up from Shins

Roll forward until ball rests under shins. Perform push-up. Keep back straight.

Prone Push-Up from Toes

Roll forward until ball rests under toes.
Perform push-up. Keep back straight.

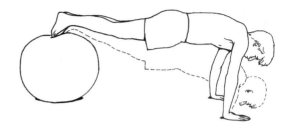

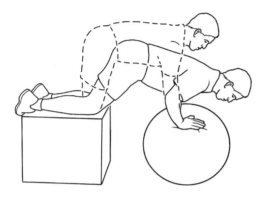

Kneeling Push-Up (Hands on Ball)

Kneel on surface level with top of ball.
Place hands on ball. Maintain shoulders
over ball. Perform a push-up.

Soccer Throw / Lunge (Standing)

Stand, holding a medicine ball behind head. Lunge step forward, throwing ball to partner. Catch ball as it returns.

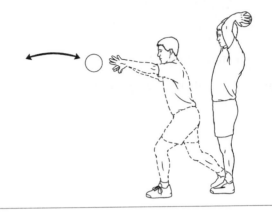

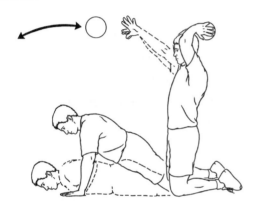

Soccer Throw / Push-Up (Kneeling)

Kneel, holding a medicine ball behind head. Throw ball forward to partner and let momentum take you to a push-up position. Push back up and catch ball as it returns.

Push-Up (Hand on Ball)

Perform push-up, one hand on medicine ball.

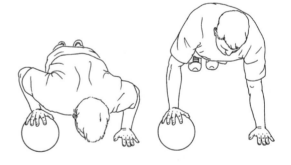

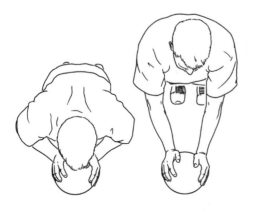

Push-Up (Hands on Ball)

Perform push-up, both hands on medicine ball.

Push-Up (Each Hand on a Ball)

Perform a push-up, each hand on medicine ball.

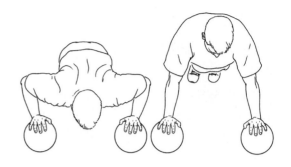

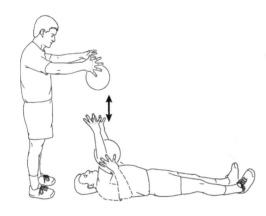

Drop / Toss

Lie on back with arms outstretched. Partner stands at head and drops a medicine ball. Catch ball with both hands. Quickly throw ball back up to partner.

Chest Pass (Half-Kneeling)

Kneel on one knee, holding a ball. Toss a medicine ball forward to partner. Catch ball as it returns.

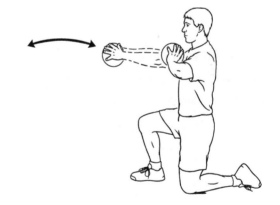

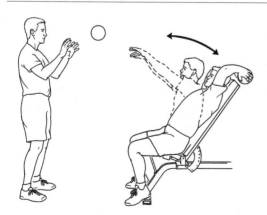

Overhead Pass (Incline Bench)

Sit holding a medicine ball behind head. Toss ball. Catch ball over head as it returns.

Shoulder Horizontal Abduction / Adduction, Elbows Straight (Aquatic)

Hold arms forward at chest level, elbows straight, thumbs up. Move arms apart, out from midline. Then move arms forward to start position.

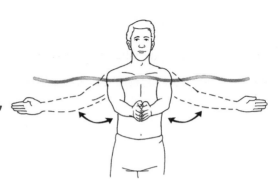

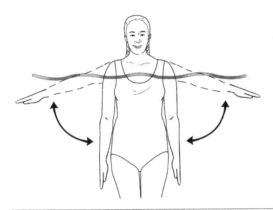

Shoulder Lateral Abduction / Adduction, Elbows Straight (Aquatic)

With arms at sides, thumbs forward, lift arms out from sides to chest height. Then pull arms down to start position.

Shoulder Forward Flexion to 90°

With arms at sides, thumbs forward, lift arms forward to chest level.

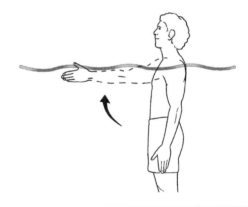

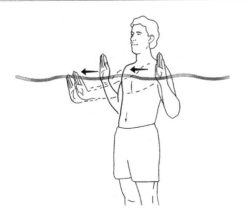

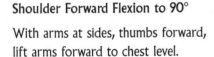

Shoulder / Elbow Forward Press (Aquatic)

Hold hands up, palms forward, elbows bent. Straighten both elbows, pushing hands forward.

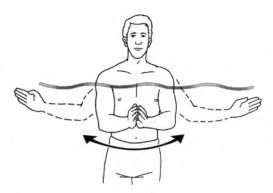

Shoulder Horizontal Fly, Elbows Bent (Aquatic)

Hold arms forward at chest level, elbow bent. Move arms apart, out from midline, keeping elbows bent.

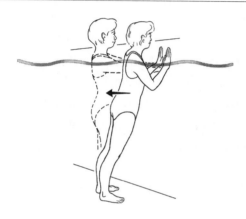

Pushaway (Aquatic)

Stand with palms on wall, elbows bent. Straighten arms, pushing away.

Chapter 2: Shoulder Exercises

The shoulder is actually a very complex structure consisting of four primary joints: the glenohumeral (ball and socket joint of the arm and the scapula), the scapulothoracic (the scapula floats on the posterior upper rib cage), the sternoclavicular (the clavicle attaches to the sternum), and the acromioclavicular (where the clavicle attaches to the anterior scapula) joints. It is the joint that has the greatest range of motion and therefore is structurally the least stable. That is, the two main parts — the glenohumeral and the scapulothoracic thoracic joints are loosely attached, the latter not having any ligaments at all. For the glenohumeral joint to move as much as it does, there are accompanying scapulothoracic, acromioclavicular, and sternoclavicular movement that must occur. Through it all, the rotator cuff muscles must work in concert with the larger agonist muscles that are pulling the humerus, or upper arm, in every which way. The main muscles are the deltoids — anterior, posterior, and middle — and the trapezius, rhomboids, pecs, and lats. Arm muscles are also involved, especially the biceps and triceps, since they actually cross the shoulder and the elbow joints.

Shoulder exercises include one or more of the following muscles: Middle Deltoid, Posterior Deltoid, Anterior Deltoid, Trapezius, Triceps, and Rhomboids.

Presses – 11 exercises
Anterior Deltoid – 9 exercises
Middle Deltoid – 8 exercises
Posterior Deltoid – 11 exercises

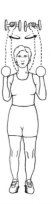

Press: Standing (Dumbbell)

Knees slightly bent, palms in, press to straight arms, rotating to palms forward at end of movement.

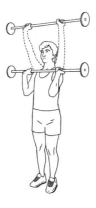

Press: Standing – Medium Grip (Barbell)

Knees slightly bent, press bar to straight arms.

Press: Behind Neck – Standing Medium Grip (Barbell)

Knees slightly bent, bar behind neck, press to straight arms, using light weights.

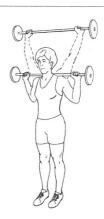

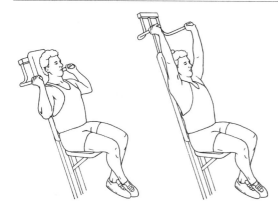

Press: Sitting (Machine)

Press handles to straight arms.

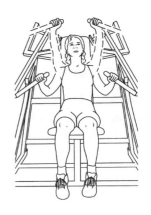

Front Deltoid Press (Machine)

Press handles to straight arms.

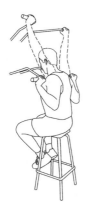

Front Deltoid Press (Machine)

Press handles to straight arms.

Press (Dumbbell)

Back straight, press dumbbells over head.

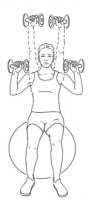

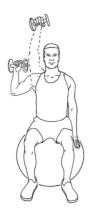

Press: Single (Dumbbell)

Back straight, press dumbbell over head. Repeat with other arm.

Press: "Arnold" (Dumbbell)

Back straight, palms facing backward, press weights over head, rotating to palms in.

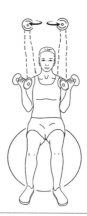

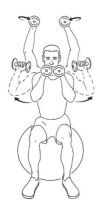

Press: "4 Point"

Palms in, elbows in, swing elbows out from sides, then press weights over head, palms forward. Rotate to palms in and return.

Press (Cable)

Back straight, press cable over head.

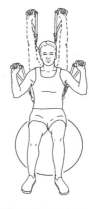

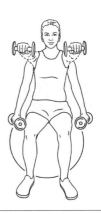

Raise: Front (Dumbbell)

Back straight, raise dumbbell forward.

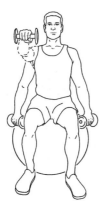

Raise: Front – Single Arm (Dumbbell)

Back straight, raise one dumbbell forward. Repeat with other arm.

Front Deltoid Raise: Single Arm (Dumbbell)

Knees slightly bent, raise dumbbell over head, keeping elbow locked. Alternate arms.

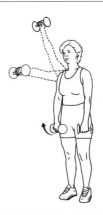

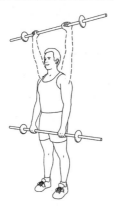

Front Deltoid Raise: Standing (Barbell)

Knees and elbows slightly bent, raise bar over head, rotating arms at shoulders only.

Front Deltoid Raise:
Standing Single Arm (Cable)

Knees and elbow slightly bent, move arm up to over head, rotating at shoulder only.

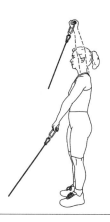

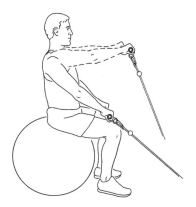

Raise: Front (Cable)

Back straight, raise cable forward.

Alphabet (Standing)

Holding medicine ball in one hand, draw the alphabet letters, first small then large.

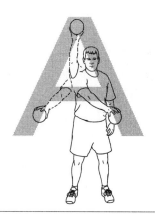

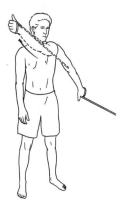

Strengthening: Resisted Diagonal

Hold tubing with arm down and out from side, thumb down. Pull arm across body and over head, rotating arm to thumb up.

Strengthening:

Resisted Diagonal Extension

Hold tubing with arm above and behind, palm up. Bring arm down across body, rotating to palm down.

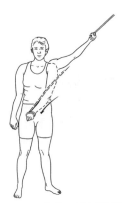

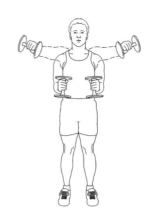

Lateral Deltoid Raise: Standing (Dumbbell)

Knees slightly bent, hold elbows at 90° angle. Raise hands and elbows level with shoulders, rotating to palms down at beginning of motion. Lead with elbows.

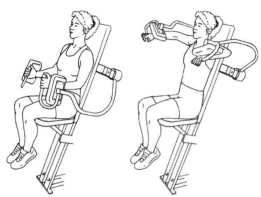

Lateral Deltoid Raise (Machine)

Arms bent 90°, raise upper arms to just above shoulder height. Lead with elbows.

Raise: Side (Cable)

Back straight, raise cable from sides.

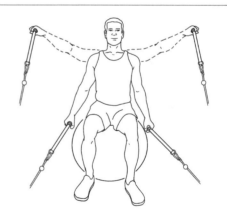

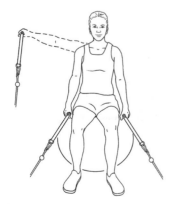

Raise: Side – Single Arm (Cable)

Back straight, raise cable from side.

Raise: Side (Dumbbell)

Back straight, raise dumbbells from sides.

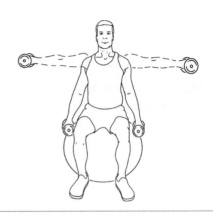

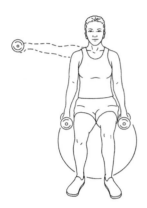

Raise: Side – Single Arm (Dumbbell)

Back straight, raise one dumbbell from side. Repeat with other arm.

Raise: Side-Lying

With trunk supported, raise dumbbell toward ceiling.

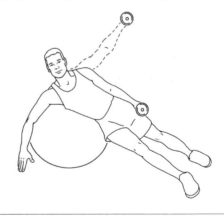

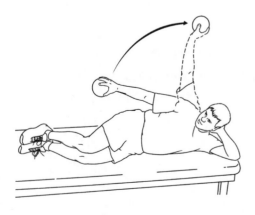

Abduction (Side-Lying)

Lie on side holding medicine ball in top hand, arm along side. Keeping arm straight, raise ball toward ceiling.

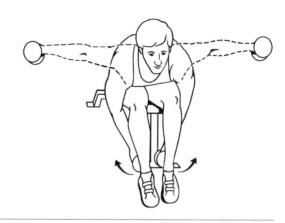

Rear Deltoid Raise: Sitting (Dumbbell)

Elbows slightly bent, palms in, raise
arms to parallel with floor.

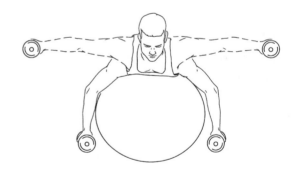

Rear Deltoid Raise: Lying (Dumbbell)

From high bench, elbows slightly bent,
palms in, raise arms to shoulder height.

Fly: Rear – Prone (Dumbbell)

Back straight, arm slightly bent, raise
dumbbells to shoulder level.

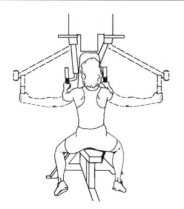

Rear Deltoid Fly (Machine)

Upper body firmly against pad, rotate
arms backward as far as possible.

Rear Deltoid Raise: Standing Single Arm (Cable)

Knees slightly bent, torso forward, back straight, raise arm to shoulder height.

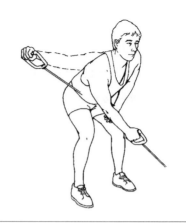

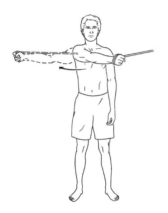

Strengthening:
Resisted Horizontal Abduction

Hold tubing in hand, elbow straight, arm in, parallel to floor. Pull arm out from side through pain-free range.

Progressive Resisted: Extension (Prone)

Holding weights, arms back, raise arms from floor, keeping elbows straight.

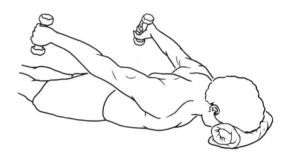

Scapular: Stabilization (Prone)

Holding weights, raise both arms out from sides. Keep elbows straight.

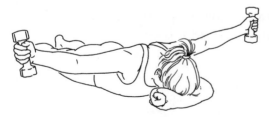

Functional Pattern Strengthening: Backhand

With feet perpendicular to anchor, and right arm across body, pull arm out from side as in tennis backhand.

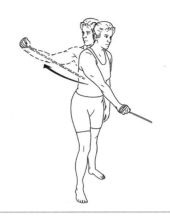

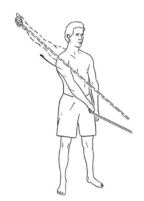

Strengthening: Resisted Diagonal

Hold tubing with arm down across body, thumb pointing back. Pull arm up and out, rotating arm to palm forward.

Strengthening: Resisted Diagonal Extension

Hold tubing with arm across body above shoulder, palm down. Gently pull down and away from body, rotating arm to palm up.

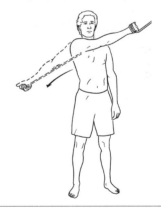

Chapter 3: Upper / Middle Back Exercises

The upper and middle back is probably the most neglected portion of the body since it can't be seen in the mirror. Yet, the development of this part of the body is critical to good posture and shoulder function. According to some authors, if we consider the weight of the head to be 10 pounds, for every inch forward that the chin projects, the neck supports that many inches x 10 pounds of weight. The added stress to the upper back muscles, throughout the day, may be cause for the stress-related headaches many in the workforce endure. Therefore, strengthening the trapezius, rhomboids, and levator scapula becomes essential for health, not just posture.

The Upper / Middle Back exercises often include one or more of the following muscles: Middle Deltoid, Posterior Deltoid, Anterior Deltoid, Trapezius, Triceps, and Rhomboids.

Tubing – 14 exercises
Dumbbells – 15 exercises
Barbells – 3 exercises
Machines – 7 exercises
Cable – 9 exercises

High Row: Standing

Face anchor, feet shoulder width apart. Palms down, pull arms back, squeezing shoulder blades together.

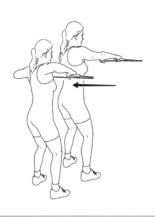

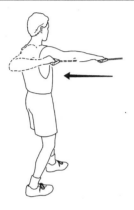

High Row: Single Arm

Face anchor in stride stance. Palm down, pull arm back while squeezing shoulder blades together.

Low Row: Single Arm

Face anchor in stride stance. Palm up, pull arm back while squeezing shoulder blades together.

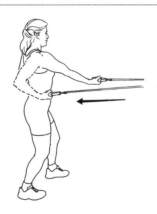

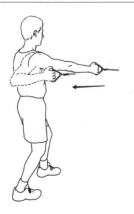

Low Row: Thumb Up (Single Arm)

Face anchor in stride stance. Thumb up, pull arm back, squeezing shoulder blades together.

Low Row: Long-Sitting

Tubing around feet and palms up, pull arms
back while squeezing shoulder blades together.

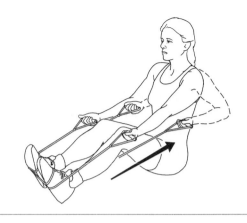

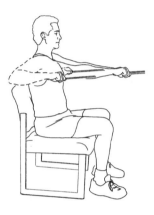

Shoulder Row: Sitting

Face anchor. Palms down, pull elbows back,
squeezing shoulder blades together.

Shoulder Row: Sitting with Trunk Flexion

Anchor tubing under feet, sitting
forward. Palms down, pull elbows back,
squeezing shoulder blades together.

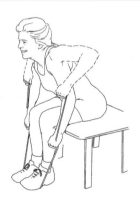

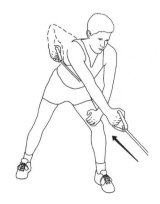

Low Row: Bent Over –
Thumb Up (Single Arm)

Face anchor in wide stride stance. Thumb up, pull
arm back, squeezing shoulder blades together.

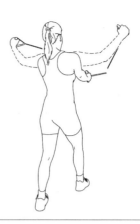

Fly: Reverse

Face anchor in stride stance, reaching forward, thumbs up. Pull arms apart and back, squeezing shoulder blades together at end position.

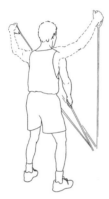

Elevation

Face anchor in shoulder width stance, arms reaching forward, thumbs up. Raise arms up and out.

Pull Down: Diagonal (Single Arm)

Side toward anchor in shoulder width stance. Arm up across body, thumb up, pull down and away.

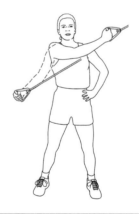

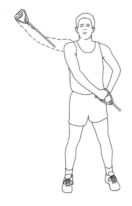

Raise: Diagonal (Single Arm)

Side toward anchor in shoulder width stance. Arm down across body, thumb up, pull up and away.

Fly: Reverse – Bent Over (Single Arm)

Side toward anchor, bend forward.
Exercising arm across body, thumb up,
pull arm out and away from body.

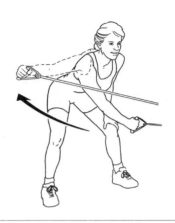

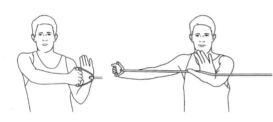

Fly: Reverse – "Dynamic Cam" (Single Arm)

Side toward anchor in shoulder width stance.
Pull arm across and away from body. Push
tubing out as exercising arm sweeps across.

Row: Bent Over – Single Arm (Dumbbell)

Lift weight to side of chest, keeping elbow close to body.

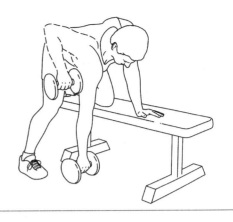

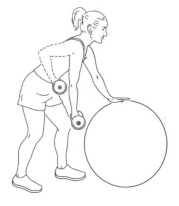

Row: Bent Over – Single Arm Reverse Grip (Dumbbell)

Using reverse grip, lift weight to side of chest, keeping elbow close to body.

Row: Single (Dumbbell)

With feet staggered, arm supported, pull weight to side of chest, keeping elbow close. Keep back straight.

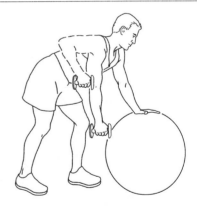

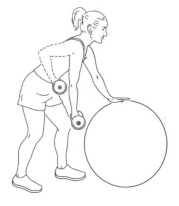

Row: Reverse Grip (Dumbbell)

With feet staggered, arm supported, pull weight to side of chest, palm forward. Keep back straight.

Row: Sitting – Bent Over (Dumbbell)

Pull weights to sides, palms facing each other.

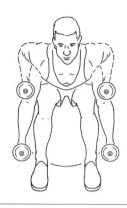

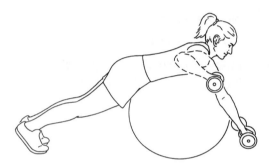

Row: Prone (Dumbbell)

Pull weights to sides, palms facing floor.

Rear Deltoid Raise: Sitting (Dumbbell)

Elbows slightly bent, palms in, raise
arms to parallel with floor.

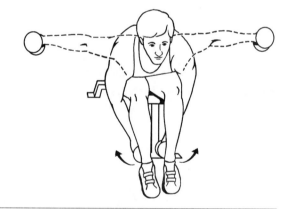

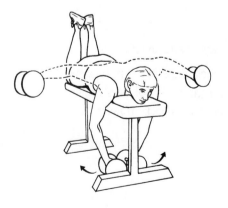

Rear Deltoid Raise: Lying (Dumbbell)

From high bench, elbows slightly bent,
palms in, raise arms to shoulder height.

Fly: Rear – Prone (Dumbbell)

Back straight, elbows slightly bent, raise dumbbells to shoulder level.

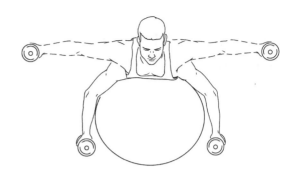

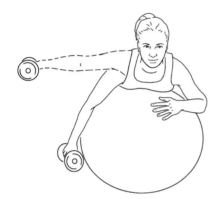

Fly: Rear – Single, Prone (Dumbbell)

Back straight, elbow slightly bent, raise one dumbbell to shoulder level. Repeat with other arm.

Row: Upright (Dumbbell)

Knees slightly bent, lift weights to chin, leading with elbows, dumbbells close together.

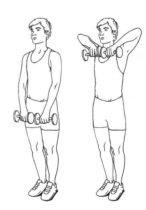

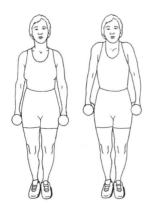

Shrug (Dumbbell)

Knees slightly bent, raise shoulders as high as possible, keeping arms straight.

Scapular: Stabilization (Prone)

Holding weights, raise both arms out from sides. Keep elbows straight. Hold.

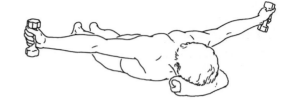

Scapular: Retraction (Prone)

Holding weights, keep arms out from sides and elbows bent. Pull elbows back, pinching shoulder blades together. Hold.

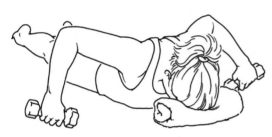

Scapular: Flexion (Prone)

Holding weights, raise arms forward. Keep elbows straight. Hold.

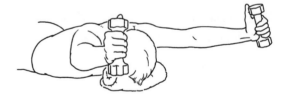

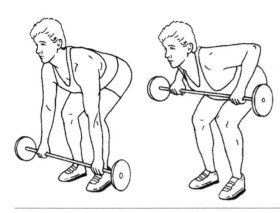

Row: Bent Over (Barbell)

Lift barbell to chest, keeping back flat and knees bent.

Row: Upright – Narrow Grip (Barbell)

Knees slightly bent, lift bar to chin, leading with elbows.

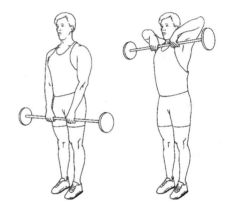

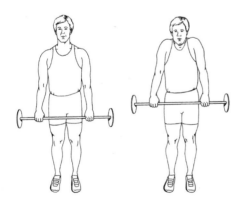

Shrug: Medium Grip (Barbell)

Knees slightly bent, raise shoulders as high as possible, keeping arms straight.

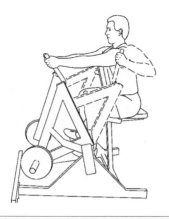

Row (Machine)

Pull handles back to sides of chest.

Row: Low (Machine)

Body firmly against pad, pull handles to torso.

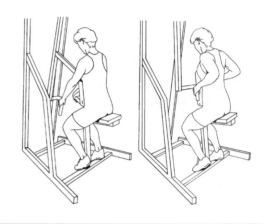

Row: High (Machine)

Body firmly against pad, pull handles to sides of chest.

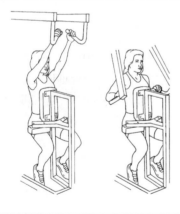

Row: Bent Over (T-Bar)

Pull handles to sides of chest, keeping back flat and knees bent.

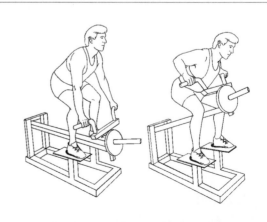

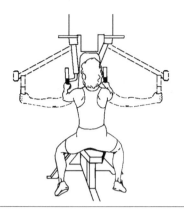

Rear Deltoid Fly (Machine)

Upper body firmly against pad, rotate arms backward as far as possible.

Row: Upright (Machine)

Knees slightly bent, pull handles up to sides of chest, leading with elbows.

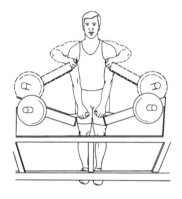

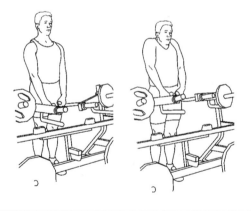

Shrug: Narrow Grip (Machine)

Knees slightly bent, raise shoulders as high as possible, keeping arms straight.

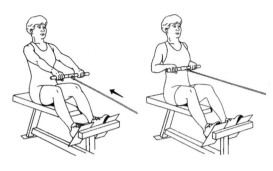

Row (Cable)

Torso erect, pull bar to lower chest.

Row: Wide Grip (Cable)

Torso erect, pull bar to chest.

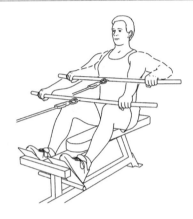

Row (V-Bar, Cable)

Torso erect, pull bar to chest.

Row: Single Arm (Cable)

Torso erect, bracing other hand on thigh, pull arm back to side of chest.

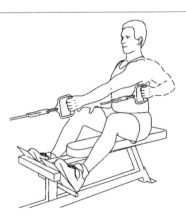

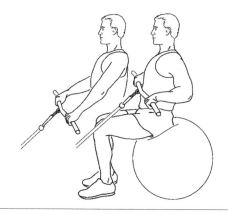

Row: Wide Grip – Sitting (Cable)

Pull weight to top of abdomen, keeping back straight.

Rear Deltoid Raise: Standing Single Arm (Cable)

Knees slightly bent, torso forward, back straight, raise arm to shoulder height.

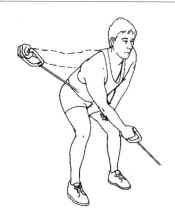

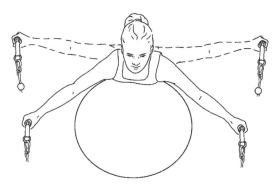

Fly: Rear – Prone (Cable)

Back straight, elbows slightly bent, raise cables in line with shoulders.

Shrug (Cable)

Knees slightly bent, raise shoulders as high as possible keeping arms straight.

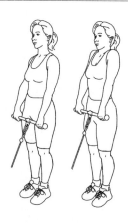

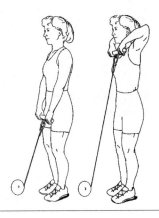

Row: Upright – Narrow Grip (Cable)

Knees slightly bent, pull bar to chin, leading with elbows.

Chapter 4: Latissimus Dorsi Exercises

The latissimus dorsi, or "lats", is the large muscle that originates from the aponeurosis of the lumbar fascia and inserts on the antero-medial upper humerus. It usually works with the teres major. Most exercises for the lats are biceps intensive, though some use triceps. Thus it has an extension moment of the lumbar spine and the shoulder. It is also an adductor of the shoulder. Finally, due to its alignment on the arm, it internally rotates the shoulder. As the largest muscle of the mid- to lower back, the lats define the shape of the back, giving the V-shape to the male athlete.

The lats are a controversial muscle in that they are often trained as adductors rather than extensors of the shoulder. Lifting lore sometimes recommends pulling the bar of a high pulley behind the neck. While there are some inherent dangers with this movement, there is little anatomical justification for this positioning. Since the lats fibers run from the posterior surface of the back to the somewhat anterior humerus, they pull from an in-front of the body position toward the origin in the back. Likewise, there are issues with how wide a grip to use to perform a pull-down movement. The only caveat here is that some arm positions may be less comfortable or less painful, depending on the status of the shoulder joints. Thus, there are few contraindicated uses of the lat exercises; in fact, some are promoting lat conditioning for those with low back problems.

Latissimus exercises include one or more of the following muscles: Middle Deltoid, Posterior Deltoid, Anterior Deltoid, Trapezius, Triceps, Biceps, Rhomboids, and Latissimus Dorsi.

Pulls – 15 exercises
Dips – 7 exercises
Sweeps – 8 exercises
Aquatic – 6 exercises

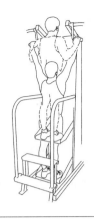

Pull-Up: Machine Assist

Pull body up until hands are even with shoulders.

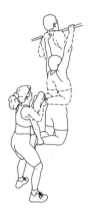

Pull-Up: Partner Assist

Partner assisting, pull body up until chin clears bar.

Pull-Up: Medium Grip

Pull body up until bar touches chin.

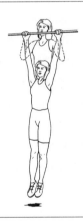

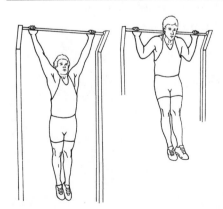

Pull-Up: Wide Grip

Pull body up until bar touches base of neck.

Pull-Up (V-Bar)

Pull body up until nose touches bar.

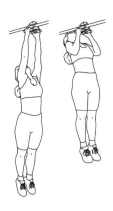

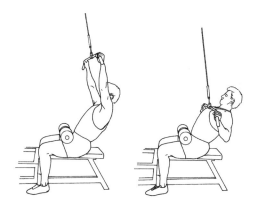

Pull-Down: 45° Angle (Cable)

Leaning back slightly, pull bar to upper chest.

Pull-Down: 45° Angle Reverse Grip (Cable)

Leaning back slightly, pull bar to upper chest.

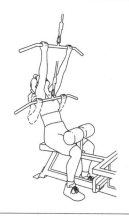

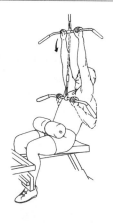

Pull-Down: 45° Angle Narrow Grip (Cable)

Leaning back slightly, pull bar to upper chest.

Pull-Down: 45° Angle (V-Bar, Cable)

Leaning back slightly, pull bar to upper chest.

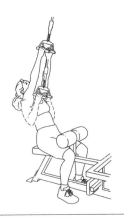

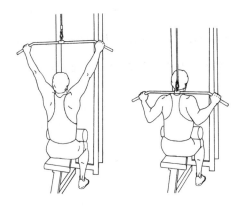

Pull-Down: Wide Grip (Cable)

Pull bar to base of neck.

Row: High (Machine)

Body firmly against pad, pull
handles to sides of chest.

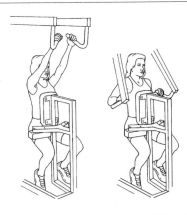

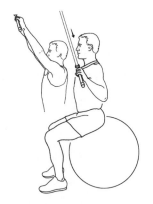

Pull-Down: Close Grip – Sitting (Cable)

Pull weight to top of chest.
Keep low back arched.

Pull-Down: Reverse Grip – Sitting (Cable)

With palms facing body, pull weight down
to top of chest. Keep low back arched.

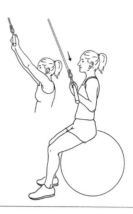

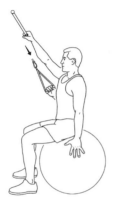

Pull-Down: Single – Sitting (Cable)

Pull weight to side of chest.
Keep low back arched.

Pull-Down: Kneeling (Cable)

Pull weight to top of chest. Keep back straight.

Caution: Spotter Advised.

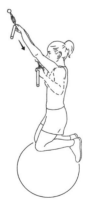

Press-Up: Sitting

Sitting on chair with palms flat on seat, slump forward a bit. Push up so bottom comes off chair.

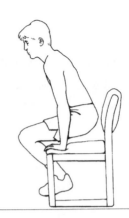

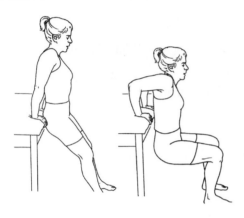

ROM: Extension

Feet shoulder width apart, holding onto table, gently lower body by bending knees until stretch is felt. Hold.

Dip (Bench)

Body almost to floor, elbows close to sides, press upward until arms are straight.

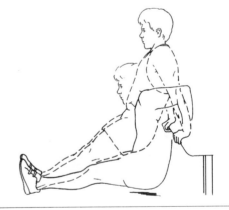

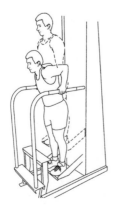

Dip: Assist (Machine)

With upper arms parallel to floor, press upward until arms are straight.

Dip (Machine)

With upper arms parallel to floor, press upward until arms are straight.

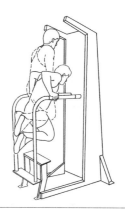

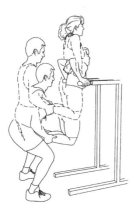

Dip: Partner Assist

Partner assisting, with upper arms parallel to floor, press upward until arms are straight.

Extension: Sitting (Machine)

Press handles downward until arms are straight.

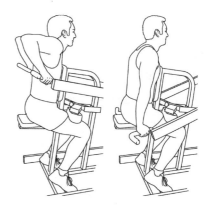

Pullover (EZ Curl Bar)

Pull bar over chest, keeping elbows
straight, trunk bridged.

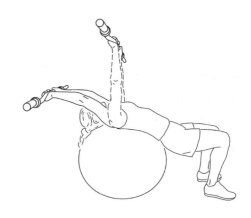

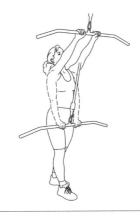

Pullover (Dumbbell)

Pull dumbbell over chest, keeping
elbows straight, trunk bridged.

Pull-Down: Standing Straight Arm, Narrow Grip (Cable)

One foot back for stability, lower
bar, keeping arms straight.

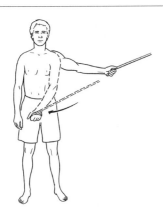

Strengthening: Resisted Adduction

Hold tubing in hand, arm out. Pull arm toward
opposite hip. Do not twist or rotate trunk.

Resistance: PNF D2 Extension

Side toward anchor in shoulder width stance:
thumb pointing back (hitchhike), pull down
across body, rotating hand and arm to palm back.

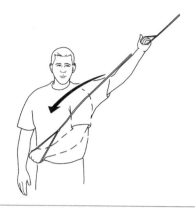

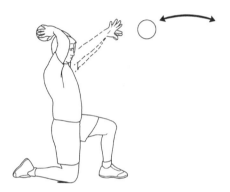

Upper Extremity: Soccer Throw (Half-Kneeling)

Kneel on one knee, holding medicine
ball behind head. Throw ball forward
to partner. Catch ball as it returns.

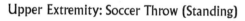

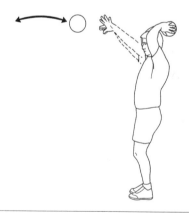

Upper Extremity: Soccer Throw (Standing)

Stand, holding medicine ball behind head. Throw
ball forward to partner. Catch ball as it returns.

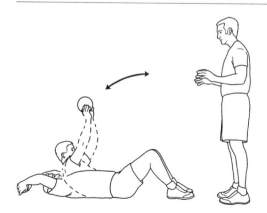

Partner Drill: Sit-Up / Ball Toss

Lie on back holding medicine ball beyond
head. Perform a sit-up and toss ball to
partner. Catch ball while returning to start.

Shoulder / Elbow Vertical Press (Aquatic)

With arms up along sides, palms down, shoulders raised and elbows bent, straighten elbows, lower shoulders, and push hands down.

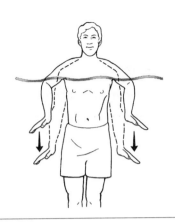

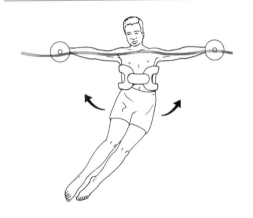

Trunk Lateral Flexion: Pendulum (Aquatic)

Swing both legs from one side to other, keeping knees straight and together. Movement should come from hips and trunk.

Shoulder Flexion / Extension, Elbows Straight: Forward / Backward Arm Swing (Aquatic)

A. Move both arms forward to water level, elbows straight, then backward past body.

B. Alternate, moving one arm forward as other arm moves backward.

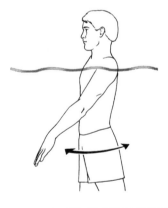

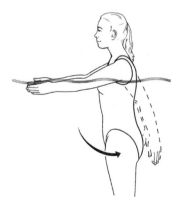

Shoulder Extension from 90° (Aquatic)

Hold arms forward at chest level, thumbs up. Pull both arms down and back.

Shoulder Lateral Abduction / Adduction, Elbows Straight (Aquatic)

With arms at sides, thumbs forward, lift both arms out from sides to chest height. Then pull arms down to start position.

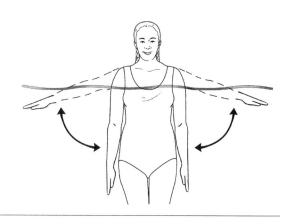

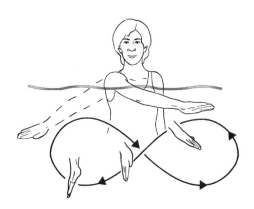

Figure Eight (Aquatic)

A. Move arm, elbow straight, in a Figure 8 pattern in front of body.
B. Arms forward, elbows straight, move arms in opposite directions in a Figure 8 pattern.

Chapter 5: Biceps Exercises

The biceps, or in weight room jargon, the "guns", flex the elbow and the shoulder. The biceps are often referred to as a single muscle but includes two others: the brachialis and the brachioradialis. The former has as its sole action the primary role of elbow flexion; that is, it is always involved. The latter is a poorly-leveraged flexor of the elbow and at the wrist. The biceps themselves have two heads — a long and short — plus attaches to the radius in a position that makes them rotate the forearm externally, or in supination. The long head is the one that acts at the shoulder. There is no evidence that the two heads can be trained separately though the influence of joint movements can affect the percent intensity that is imposed on the biceps. They are sometimes a source of pain and injury to the shoulder, but are usually trained without much concern for joint safety. Obviously, when caution is warranted, just reduced loads and restricting certain ranges will be sufficient. Otherwise, most of the movements for the biceps require elbow flexion.

Biceps exercises include one or more of the following muscles: Biceps Brachii, Brachialis, Brachioradialis, Latissimus Dorsi, Trapezius, and Anterior Deltoid.

Pulls – 4 exercises
Dumbbells – 13 exercises
Barbells – 7 exercises
Machines / Cable – 8 exercises
Tubing – 3 exercises

Pull-Down: 45° Angle (Cable)

Leaning back slightly, pull bar to upper chest.

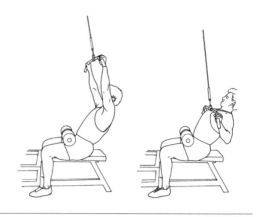

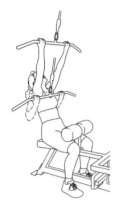

Pull-Down: 45° Angle Reverse Grip (Cable)

Leaning back slightly, pull bar to upper chest.

Pull-Up: Medium Grip

Pull body up until bar touches chin.

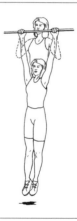

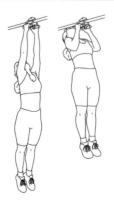

Pull-Up (V-Bar)

Pull body up until nose touches bar.

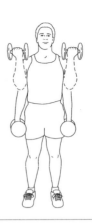

Curl: Standing (Dumbbell)

Knees slightly bent, hold weights at sides, palms in. Curl arms toward shoulders, rotating to palms up while beginning curl.

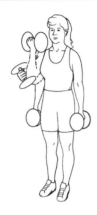

Curl: Standing Alternating (Dumbbell)

Knees slightly bent, hold weights at sides, palms in. Curl arm toward shoulder rotating to palm up while beginning curl. Alternate arms.

Curl: Standing Inner Biceps (Dumbbell)

Knees slightly bent, hold weights at sides, palms forward. Curl arms toward shoulders, rotating to palms out while beginning curl. Keep forearms in line with sides of torso.

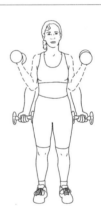

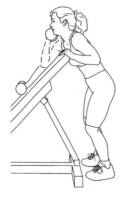

Curl: Standing Single Arm – Incline (Dumbbell)

Curl arm toward shoulder, keeping upper arm in contact with bench.

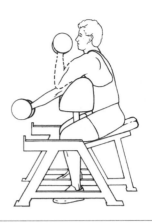

Curl: Sitting – Single Arm
(Preacher Bench, Dumbbell)

Curl arm toward side of shoulder, keeping upper arm in contact with bench.

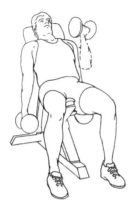

Curl: Sitting Incline –
Alternating (Dumbbell)

Hold weights at sides, palms in. Curl arm toward shoulder, rotating to palm up while beginning curl. Alternate arms.

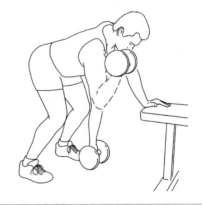

Curl: Standing Single Arm –
Concentration (Dumbbell)

Curl arm to shoulder, keeping upper arm perpendicular to floor.

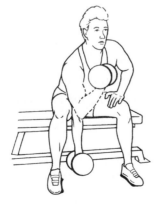

Curl: Sitting Single Arm –
Concentration (Dumbbell)

Curl arm toward shoulder, bracing upper arm against inner thigh and keeping upper arm perpendicular to floor.

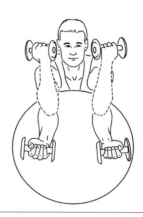

Curl: Preacher (Dumbbell)

Kneel over ball with elbows fully
extended. Curl dumbbells.

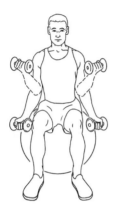

Curl (Dumbbell)

Supported by ball with knees bent,
palms forward, curl dumbbells. Do
not allow shoulder to flex.

Curl: Hammer Grip (Dumbbell)

Supported by ball with knees slightly bent,
forearms neutral, palms in, curl dumbbells.

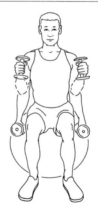

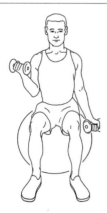

Curl: Alternating (Dumbbell)

Supported by ball with knees slightly bent,
curl one dumbbell. Repeat with other arm.

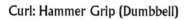

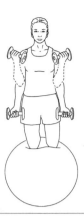

Curl: Kneeling (Dumbbell)

Kneel on ball with elbows fully extended. Curl dumbbells.

Curl: Standing – Narrow Grip (Barbell)

Knees slightly bent, curl arms toward shoulders.

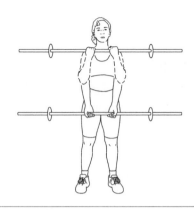

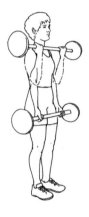

Curl: Standing Medium Grip (Barbell)

Knees slightly bent, curl arms toward shoulders.

Curl: Standing Narrow Grip (EZ Curl Bar)

Knees slightly bent, curl arms toward shoulders.

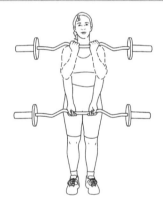

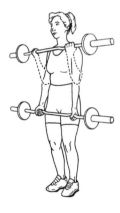

Curl: Standing Medium Grip
(EZ Curl Bar)

Knees slightly bent, curl arms toward shoulders.

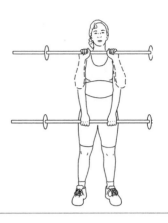

Curl: Standing – Narrow Reverse Grip (Barbell)

Knees slightly bent, using narrow reverse grip, curl arms toward shoulders.

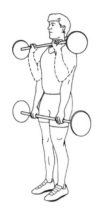

Curl: Standing Medium Reverse Grip (Barbell)

Knees slightly bent, using medium reverse grip, curl arms toward shoulders.

Curl: Sitting – Medium Grip
(Preacher Bench, EZ Curl Bar)

Curl arms toward shoulders.

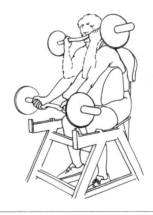

Curl: Standing (Cable)

Knees slightly bent, curl arms toward shoulders, keeping upper arms close to sides.

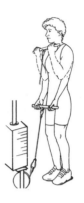

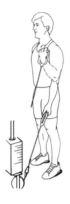

Curl: Standing Single Arm (Cable)

Knees slightly bent, curl arm toward shoulder, keeping upper arm close to side.

Curl: Standing (Cable)

Knees slightly bent, curl arms toward shoulders, keeping upper arms parallel with floor.

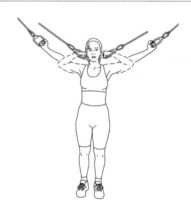

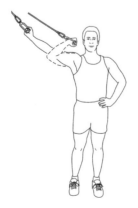

Curl: Standing Single Arm (Cable)

Knees slightly bent, curl arm toward shoulder, keeping upper arm parallel to floor.

Curl: Preacher (Cable)

Kneel over ball, elbows fully extended. Curl cable.

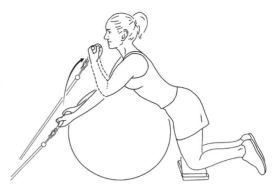

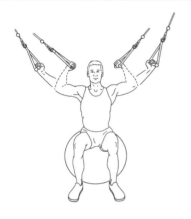

Curl: Sitting (Cable – High Pulley)

Grasp handles with elbows fully extended and upper arm parallel to floor. Curl cables.

Curl: Sitting (Cable – Low Pulley)

Grasp handles, elbows fully extended, upper arm parallel to floor. Curl cables.

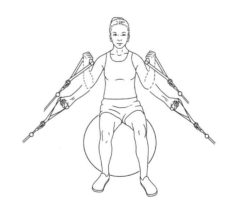

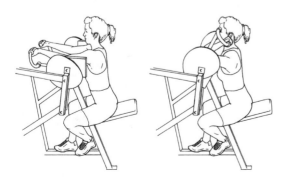

Curl: Sitting (Machine)

Wrists straight, curl arms toward shoulders, keeping upper arms in contact with pad.

Curl: Standing

Anchor tubing under front foot in stride stance. Palms forward, curl arms.

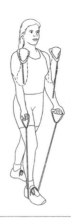

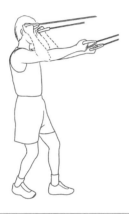

Curl: Standing – Elevated

Face anchor in stride stance. With arms reaching forward, palms up, curl arms.

Curl: Palm Up (Single Arm)

Anchor tubing under back foot in stride stance. Palm up, curl arm toward shoulder.

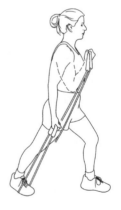

Chapter 6: Triceps Exercises

The triceps are the muscles on the back of the upper arm. There are three origins of the triceps; one of them — the long head — is from the scapula, giving it the ability to extend the shoulder and the elbow. The other two heads affect only the elbow. The triceps are used for all pushing movements, whether off the chest or from the shoulders. At the shoulder, since it does extend it, the triceps are actually used in some pulling movements, but these movements are not used for training them.

Triceps exercises include one or more of the following muscles: Triceps, Posterior Deltoid, Pectoralis Major, and Latissimus Dorsi.

Push-Ups / Press — 4 exercises
Dips — 6 exercises
Dumbbells — 9 exercises
Barbells — 9 exercises
Tubing — 8 exercises
Machines / Cable — 12 exercises

Push-Up Plus: Diamond

Place thumbs and forefingers together. Balance on toes. Perform a push-up. Give an extra push at end to bring shoulder blades forward on rib cage.

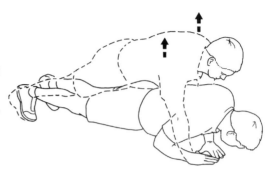

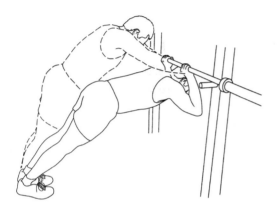

Extension: Leaning

Hold head under bar and forearms perpendicular to floor. Press to straight arms, keeping feet stationary.

Push-Up: Close Grip – Kneeling

With hands close, extend elbows by pushing away from ball. Keep back straight.

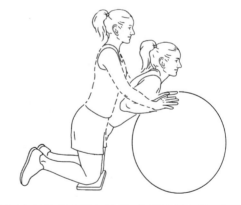

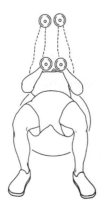

Press: Close Grip – Supine (Dumbbell)

Hold dumbbells over chest, elbows in close. Extend elbows.

Dip (Bench)

Body almost to floor, elbows close to sides, press upward until arms are straight.

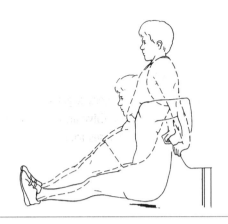

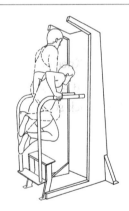

Dip: Assist (Machine)

With upper arms parallel to floor, press upward until arms are straight.

Dip (Machine)

With upper arms parallel to floor, press upward until arms are straight

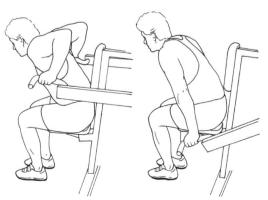

Extension: Sitting (Machine)

Press handles downward until arms are straight.

Extension: Sitting (Machine)

Press handles downward until arms are straight.

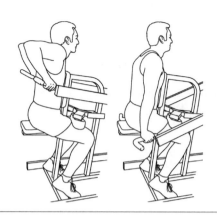

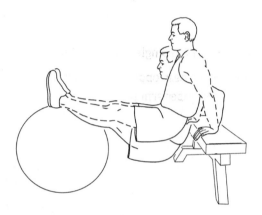

Dip: Feet on Ball

With feet supported by ball and hands firmly on bench, extend elbows while tightening triceps.

Kickback: Bent Over – Single Arm (Dumbbell)

Straighten arm, keeping upper
arm in line with body.

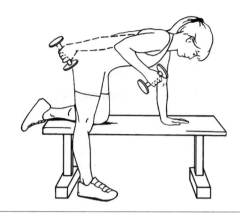

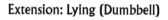

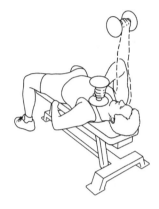

Extension: Lying – Single Arm (Dumbbell)

Hold dumbbell near opposite shoulder. Straighten
arm, keeping upper arm perpendicular to floor.

Extension: Lying (Dumbbell)

Straighten arms, keeping upper
arms perpendicular to floor.

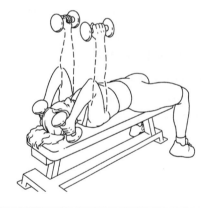

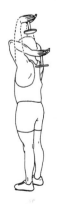

Extension: Standing (Dumbbell)

Knees slightly bent, straighten arms, keeping
upper arms close to sides of head.

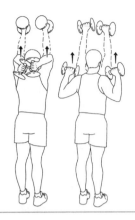

Extension / Press: Standing (Dumbbell)

Knees slightly bent, straighten arms, keeping upper arms close to sides of head, palms in. Rotating palms forward, lower weights to shoulders then press to straight arms. Repeat sequence each repetition.

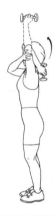

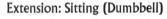

Extension: Standing – Single Arm (Dumbbell)

Knees slightly bent, straighten arm, using other hand to keep upper arm stable.

Extension: Sitting (Dumbbell)

With upper arms vertical, raise dumbbell by extending elbows. Keep feet flat and back straight.

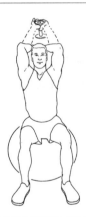

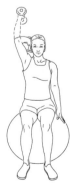

Extension: Single – Sitting (Dumbbell)

With upper arm vertical, raise dumbbell by extending elbow. Keep feet flat and back straight. Repeat with other arm.

Extension: Supine (Dumbbell)

Bridge trunk, head and neck supported, upper arms vertical. Raise dumbbells by extending elbows.

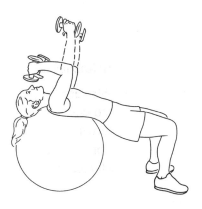

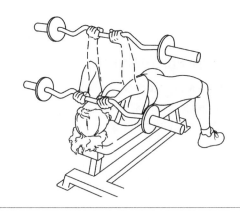

Extension: Lying – Narrow Grip (EZ Curl Bar)

Hold bar just off forehead. Straighten arms, keeping elbows as close together as possible.

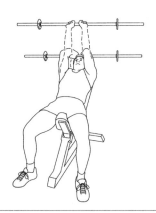

Extension: Lying – Narrow Grip (Barbell)

Hold bar just off forehead. Straighten arms, keeping elbows as close together as possible.

Extension: Sitting, Incline – Narrow Grip (Barbell)

Hold bar just off top of head. Straighten arms, keeping elbows as close together as possible.

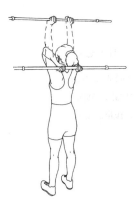

Extension: Standing – Narrow Grip (Barbell)

Knees slightly bent, straighten arms, keeping upper arms close to sides of head.

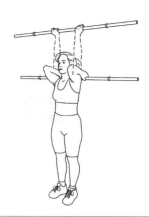

Extension: Standing – Reverse Grip (Barbell)

Knees slightly bent, using reverse
grip, straighten arms.

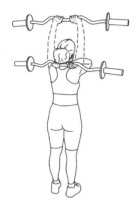

Extension: Standing – Narrow Grip (EZ Curl Bar)

Knees slightly bent, straighten arms, keeping
upper arms close to side of head.

Press: Close Grip – Supine (EZ Curl Bar)

Hold bar over chest with elbows
in close. Extend elbows.

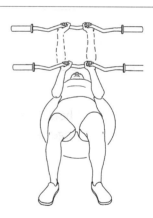

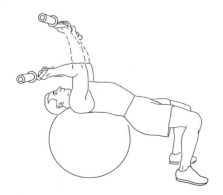

Extension: Supine (EZ Curl Bar)

Bridge trunk, head and neck supported,
upper arms vertical grasping bar.
Raise bar by extending elbows.

Extension: Supine (Barbell)

Bridge trunk, head and neck supported,
upper arms vertical grasping bar.
Raise bar by extending elbows.

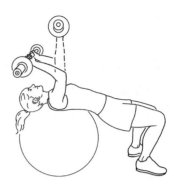

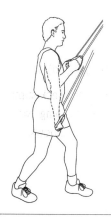

Press: Standing

Face anchor in stride stance. Thumbs up, straighten arms, rotating to palms down.

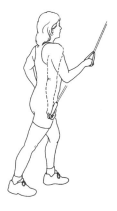

Press: Standing – Pronation (Single Arm)

Face anchor in slight stride stance. Palm down, straighten arm, maintaining hand position.

Press: Standing – Supination (Single Arm)

Face anchor in slight stride stance. Palm up, straighten arm, maintaining hand position.

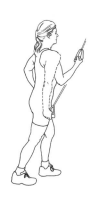

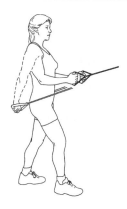

Press: Standing – Backward

Face anchor in stride stance. Thumbs up, press arms backward, rotating to palms back.

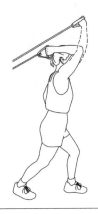

Press: Standing – Over Head (Single Arm)

Face away from anchor in stride stance. Straighten arm to palm forward.

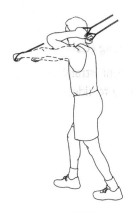

Press: Standing – Forward

Face away from anchor in stride stance. Thumbs down, press arms forward, rotating to palms down.

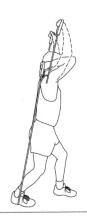

Press: Standing – Over Head

In stride stance, tubing anchored under back foot, grasp handles behind head. Thumbs down, straighten arms, rotating to palms forward.

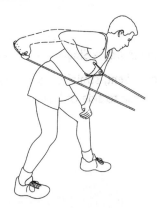

Kick-Back: Single Arm

Face anchor in wide stride stance. Support trunk with free hand on knee. Thumb up, extend arm backward.

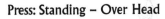

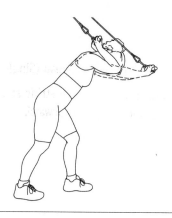

Extension: Standing (Cable)

One leg forward for balance, straighten arms, keeping elbows close to sides of head.

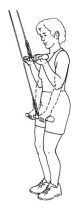

Extension: Standing (Cable)

Knees slightly bent, straighten arms, keeping upper arms close to sides of body.

Extension: Standing (Cable)

Knees slightly bent, straighten arms, keeping upper arms close to ears.

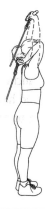

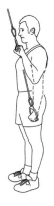

Extension: Standing – Single Arm (Cable)

Knees slightly bent, straighten arm, keeping upper arm close to side of body.

Extension: Standing – Single Arm (Cable)

Knees slightly bent, straighten arm, using other hand to keep upper arm stable.

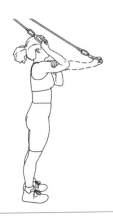

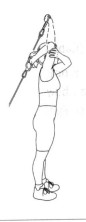

Extension: Standing – Single Arm (Cable)

Knees slightly bent, straighten arm, using other hand to keep upper arm stable.

Extension: Sitting – Single Arm (Cable)

Straighten arm, keeping upper arm close to side of body.

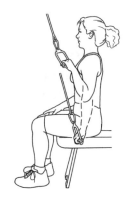

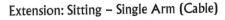

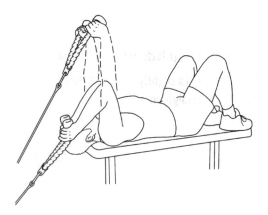

Extension: Lying (Rope Grip)

Straighten arms, keeping upper arms as close together as possible and perpendicular to floor.

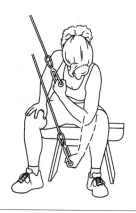

Extension: Sitting – Single Arm Concentration (Cable)

Straighten arm, bracing elbow against knee.

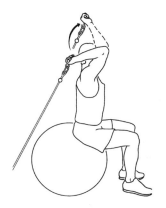

Extension: Sitting (Cable)

With upper arms vertical, raise cable by extending elbows. Keep feet flat and back straight.

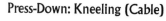

Press-Down: Kneeling (Cable)

Grasp handle and kneel on ball. Press cable. Keep back straight.

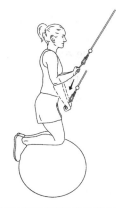

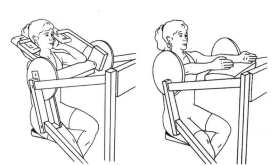

Extension: Sitting (Machine)

Sit with shoulders slightly higher than support pad. Straighten arms.

Chapter 7: Abdominal Exercises

The abdominals, or abs, are the superficial muscles of the anterior lower torso that flex and rotate the spine. They originate on the pelvis and insert on the ribs. As such, they pull the ribs forward when the pelvis is stable, and the pelvis is pulled into a posterior tilt when the upper trunk is stable. The two external layers of the abdominal wall are under more voluntary control whereas the deepest layer, the transverse abdominis (TVA), is a more reflex-based ab muscle that neither is visible nor involved in moving the spine. The TVA, whose fibers run horizontally around the abdomen like a corset, has been demonstrated to be a primary spinal stabilizer via its attachment to the thoracolumbar fascia in the back and its anticipatory contraction prior to movement of an extremity. Due to its lack of visibility and mobilizing ability, the TVA exercises are not included in this chapter.

The primary spinal flexor is the rectus abdominis (RA), otherwise known as the six-pack, for those lean and hypertrophied enough for the separations of this muscle to be visible. The tendinous inscription that bisects the length of the muscle — the linea alba — and the 2-3 horizontal divisions that separate the muscle into 6-8 smaller units do not define the muscles actions, only its appearance. The concept of lower and upper abs is debatable. What is known is that the firing of the motor nerve that feeds the RA causes the entire muscle to contract. Where the exerciser "feels" the muscle contraction varies according to the positions and motions that are occurring as a result of the contraction of the entire muscle. Its attachment to the symphysis pubis and the mid-line of the middle to lower ribs puts it in an optimal position to flex the spine from either end, the pelvis or the trunk.

The bilateral external and internal obliques operate both as bilateral structures and unilaterally. The external oblique's (EO) fibers run diagonally from the midline of the trunk toward the lateral aspect of the pelvis. When both sides of the EO fire, they exert a spinal flexion moment that assists the RA. The internal oblique's (IO) fibers run diagonally from the lateral rib cage toward the medial rim of the ilium. Together they also pull the spine into flexion. It is when the EO and IO on one side contract that they bend the spine laterally toward that side. When the EO on the right and the IO on the left contract, spinal rotation occurs toward the left; likewise the left EO with the right IO turn the trunk to the right. Against a heavy resistance, the five muscles of the anterior abdominal wall — the RA and the left and right IO and EO — work together to help flex the spine.

Many ab exercises have a hip flexion component, either requiring the hips to be held in flexion or to actually flex while controlling against lumbar extension. The anterior location of the hip flexor, the iliopsoas, on the lumbar vertebrae directs a lordotic pull on the lumbar spine during high resistance hip flexion. Ab exercises that have a hip flexion moment are safe only if the abs can control against this lordotic tension; this is a back-flattening move that, when it weakens, allows the spine to arch.

Abdominal exercises include one or more of the following muscles: Rectus Abdominis, External Obliquus, Internal Obliquus, Transverse Abdominis, Iliopsoas.

> Calisthenics — 22 exercises
> Machines / Weights — 10 exercises
> Stability Balls — 11 exercises
> Tubing — 4 exercises
> Medicine Balls — 10 exercises

Crunch: Bent Knee

Arms straight, tighten abdominals, raise
shoulders and upper back toward ceiling.
Keep head and neck in line with spine.
Keep low and middle back on floor.

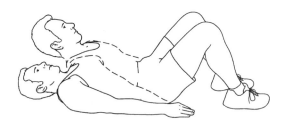

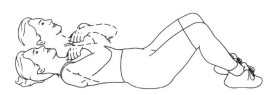

Crunch: Bent Knee

Arms crossed, tighten abdominals, raise
shoulders and upper back toward ceiling.
Keep head and neck in line with spine.
Keep low and middle back on floor.

Crunch: Bent Knee

Arms behind head, tighten abdominals, raise
shoulders and upper back toward ceiling.
Keep head and neck in line with spine.
Keep low and middle back on floor.

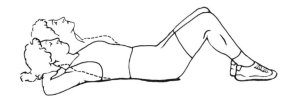

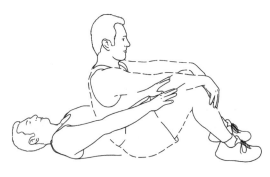

Sit-Up: Bent Knee

Arms straight, tighten abdominals, bend at
waist, curling upper body toward knees.

Sit-Up: Bent Knee

Arms crossed, tighten abdominals, bend at waist, curling upper body toward knees.

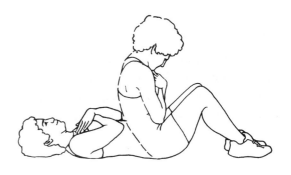

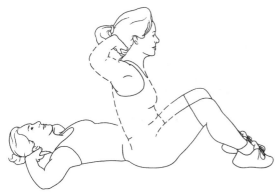

Sit-Up: Bent Knee

Hands at head, tighten abdominals, bend at waist, curling upper body toward knees.

Crunch: Raised Leg

Arms straight, legs up, bent, ankles crossed, tighten abdominals, raise shoulders and upper back toward ceiling. Keep head and neck in line with spine. Keep low and middle back on floor.

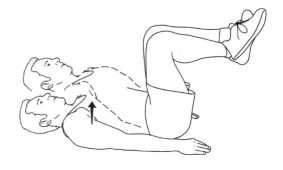

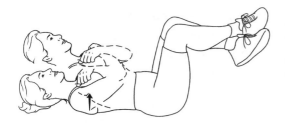

Crunch: Raised Leg

Arms crossed, legs up, bent, ankles crossed, tighten abdominals, raise shoulders and upper back toward ceiling. Keep head and neck in line with spine. Keep low and middle back on floor.

Crunch: Raised Leg

Hands at head, legs up, bent, ankles crossed, tighten abdominals, raise shoulders and upper back toward ceiling. Keep head and neck in line with spine. Keep low and middle back on floor.

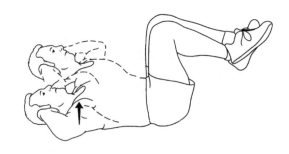

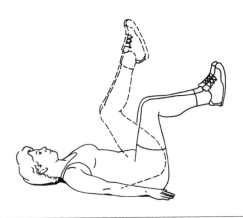

Crunch: Reverse

With knees at 90° angle, tighten abdominals, curl hips up until low back clears floor.

Sit-Up: Twist – Bent Leg

One ankle across other knee, tighten abdominals, twist upper body to touch opposite elbow to knee.

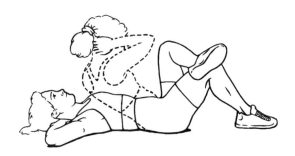

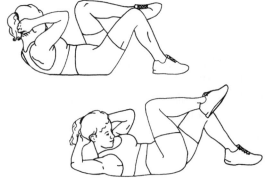

Crunch: Twist – Bent Leg, Alternating

Legs bent, tighten abdominals, raise upper body and one leg. Twist to touch opposite elbow to raised knee. Alternate sides.

Sit-Up: Three-Quarter – Straight Leg

Arms straight, tighten abdominals, raise upper body three-quarters of the way to perpendicular with floor. Keep back straight.

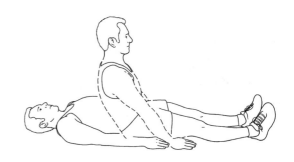

Sit-Up: Three-Quarter – Straight Leg

Arms crossed, tighten abdominals, raise upper body three-quarters of the way to perpendicular with floor. Keep back straight.

Sit-Up: Three-Quarter – Straight Leg

Hands at head, tighten abdominals, raise upper body three-quarters of the way to perpendicular with floor. Keep back straight.

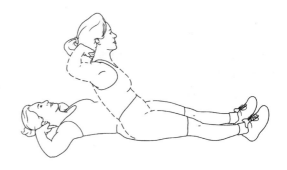

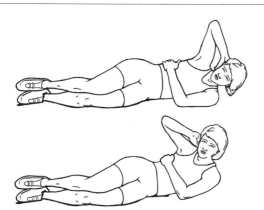

Crunch: Side

With knees bent, tighten abdominals, flex upper body upward, moving elbow toward hip.

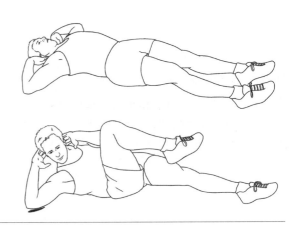

Crunch: Scissor Kick / Twist

Tighten abdominals, raise upper body, twist to side, touching elbow to opposite raised knee. Alternate sides.

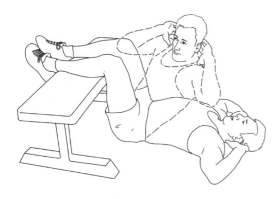

Sit-Up: Twist – Bent Knee

Tighten abdominals, twist upper body, touching elbow to inside of opposite knee. Alternate sides.

Knee Raise: Sitting

Tighten abdominals, and bend legs, pulling knees toward chest.

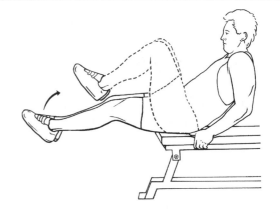

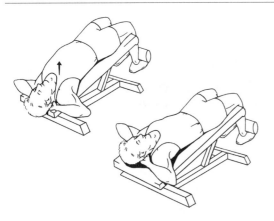

Crunch: Decline

Tighten abdominals, raise shoulders and upper back toward ceiling, keeping head and neck in line with spine. Keep low and middle back on bench.

Sit-Up: Twist – Decline

Arms crossed on chest, tighten abdominals, raise upper body, twisting to side. Keep back straight. Alternate sides.

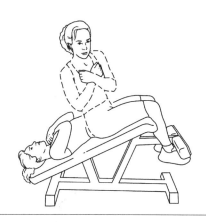

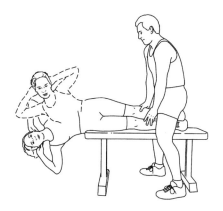

Hyperextension: Side – Partner Assist

Partner stabilizes legs. Upper body bent at waist toward floor, tighten abdominals, flex upward as far as possible.

Knee Raise

Tighten abdominals and bend legs,
pulling knees toward chest.

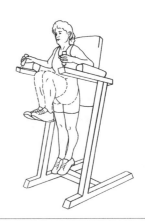

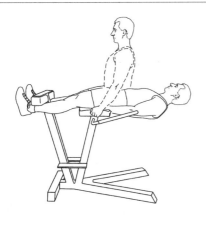

Sit-Up (Roman Chair)

Upper body parallel to floor,
tighten abdominals, sit up.

Hyperextension: Side

Body bent at waist to side, tighten abdominals,
bring upper body up, in line with legs.

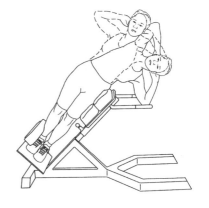

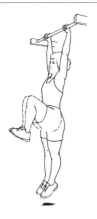

Knee Raise: Hanging

Tighten abdominals and bend legs,
pulling knees toward chest.

Knee Raise: Hanging

Tighten abdominals and bend legs, pulling knees toward chest.

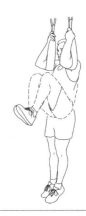

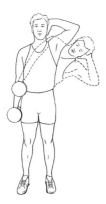

Side Bend (Dumbbell)

Tighten abdominals and bend to side as far as possible.

Side Bend (Cable)

Tighten abdominals and bend to side as far as possible.

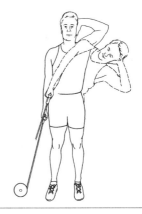

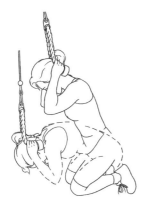

Crunch (Cable)

Tighten abdominals and curl upper body downward moving elbows toward knees.

Abdominal Wheel

Tighten abdominals and roll out without allowing upper body or arms to touch ground. Return to starting position.

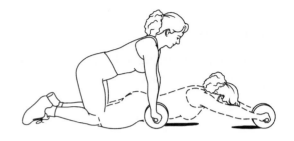

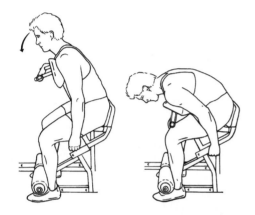

Crunch: Sitting (Machine)

Chest against pad, tighten abdominals and curl upper body toward knees.

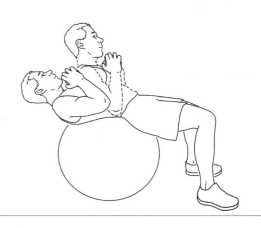

Crunch (Dumbbell)

Hold dumbbell on upper chest, low back supported. Tighten abdominals by bringing ribs toward pelvis until shoulders clear ball.

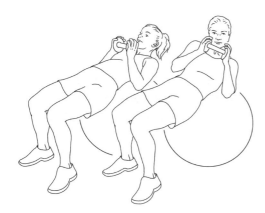

Crunch: Alternating (Dumbbell)

Hold dumbbell on upper chest, low back supported. Tighten abdominals by bringing right ribs toward left pelvis. Repeat to other side.

Crunch (Cable)

Grasp rope handle, low back supported. Tighten abdominals by bringing ribs toward pelvis until shoulders clear ball.

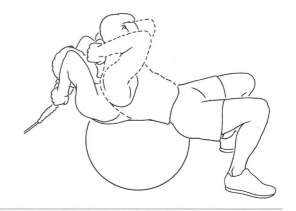

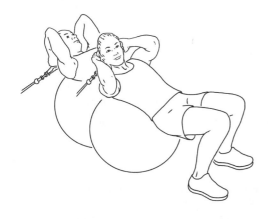

Crunch: Alternating (Cable)

Grasp rope handle, low back supported. Tighten abdominals by bringing left ribs toward right pelvis until shoulder clears ball. Repeat to other side.

Twist: Supine (Dumbbell)

Bridge trunk, head, neck, and shoulders supported, arms extended over head holding dumbbell. Rotate trunk to the right, keeping arms extended. Repeat to other side.

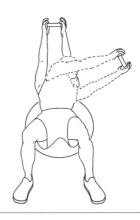

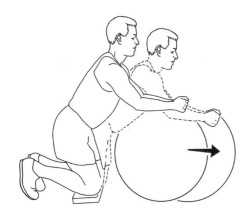

Ball Roll: Basic

With forearms on ball and back straight, begin to roll forward, progressively tensing abdominals. Breathing out, roll back to start position.

Caution: Do not hyperextend low back.

Ball Roll: Intermediate

With hands on ball and back straight, begin to roll forward, progressively tensing abdominals.

Caution: Do not hyperextend low back.
Breathing out, roll back to start position.

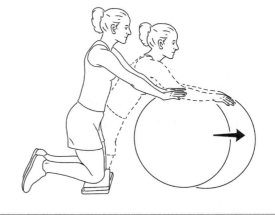

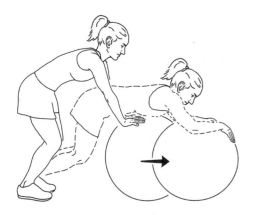

Ball Roll: Advanced

With hands on ball, back straight, knees off the floor, begin to roll forward, progressively tensing abdominals.

Caution: Do not hyperextend the low back.
Breathing out, roll back to start position.

Ball Roll: Prop on Forearms (Gymball)

Prop on ball with elbows under shoulders. Keep back straight. Roll ball forward and backward.

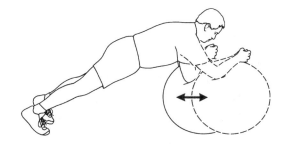

Ball Walk to Thighs with Hip Extension (Prone)

Walk forward on ball until it rests under thighs. Raise one thigh from ball. Return. Repeat with other thigh.

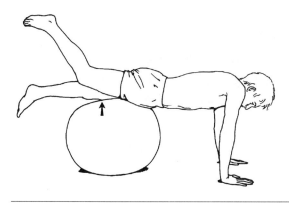

Ball Walk to Toes with Hip Extension (Prone)

Walk forward on ball until it rests under toes. Raise one leg from ball. Return. Repeat with other leg.

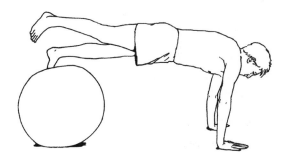

Twist: Standing

Side toward anchor in wide stance, reach toward anchor. Thumbs up, pull away from anchor. Keep arm furthest from anchor straight.

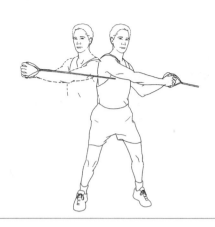

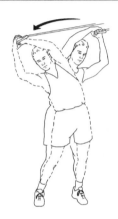

Side Bend: Standing

Side toward anchor in wide stance, arms above head, tilt trunk toward anchor. Grasp handle and pull away from anchor.

Chop: Standing – Diagonal

Side toward anchor in wide stance, reach up toward anchor. Thumbs up, pull down and away from anchor.

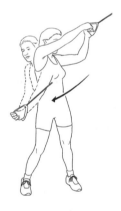

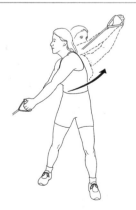

Pull: Standing – Diagonal

Side toward anchor in wide stride stance, reach down toward anchor. Thumbs up, arms straight, pull up and away.

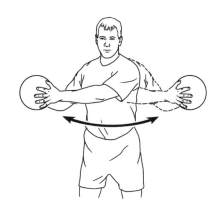

Chop: Rotational (Medicine Ball)

Hold medicine ball with arms straight. Quickly rotate ball from side to side.

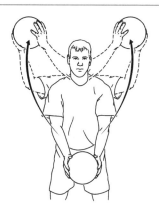

Circle (Medicine Ball)

Hold medicine ball with arms straight. Rapidly move arms in circle counterclockwise.

Chop: V (Medicine Ball)

Hold medicine ball to chest. Quickly move arms in V shape: up and out, then down, then up and out on other side.

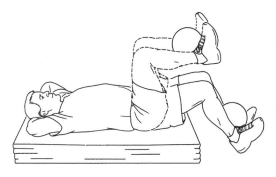

Curl: Reverse – Supine (Medicine Ball)

Lie on back, holding medicine ball between feet, knees bent 90°. Lift knees toward chest.

Curl / Crunch: Reverse – Supine (Medicine Ball)

Lie on back, holding medicine ball between feet, knees bent 90°. Lift knees toward chest while lifting upper body.

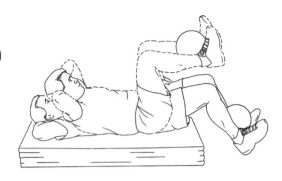

Curl: Reverse – V Sitting on Mat (Medicine Ball)

Sit on mat, holding medicine ball between feet, knees straight. Lean back from hips and hold. Lift knees toward chest.

Sit-Up (Medicine Ball))

Holding medicine ball to chest, tighten abdominals, sit up.

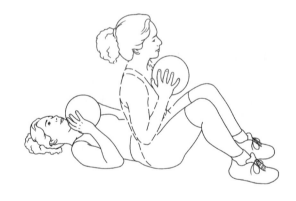

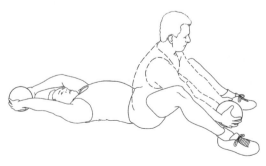

Sit-Up (Medicine Ball)

Holding medicine ball beyond head, tighten abdominals, sit up, touching ball to floor between feet.

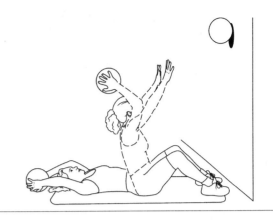

Sit-Up: Wall Throw (Medicine Ball)

Holding medicine ball beyond head, tighten abdominals, sit up and bounce ball off wall.

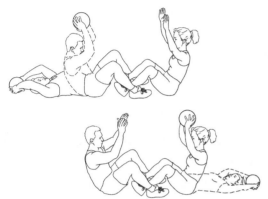

Catch (Medicine Ball)

Interlock legs. Tighten abdominals and alternate sit-up motions with partner while gently tossing ball to each other.

Chapter 8: Low Back Exercises

The muscles of the low back are often emphasized in isolation in the weight room but not in the clinic. The ones that span the vertebrae are trained in most low back exercises in the fitness arena. From a therapeutic perspective, the pronounced role of the abdominals, especially the TVA, are included in a low back program. Even the pelvic muscles are addressed. For the purposes of this book, the low back exercises will include those exercises that are specific and general, if they emphasize those muscles of the lumbar spine. As such we will address those in the posterior lower trunk in this chapter.

The muscles are divisible into two basic groups, intrinsic and extrinsic. The intrinsic muscles are those that connect 2 – 4 vertebrae to each other, such as the multifidus and intertransversarii. The extrinsic muscles tend to lie laterally to the vertebrae's midline and attach more than two together. The iliocostalis lumborum, the longissimus, and the spinalis thoracis are more superficial and span several vertebrae. They are better positioned to act bilaterally as extensors or unilaterally as lateral flexors or rotators. These longer, larger muscles constitute the erector spinae. The other important low back muscle is the quadratus lumborum (QL). This attaches from the iliac crest to the lumbar vertebrae and last rib on each side. Unilaterally, the QL tilts the spine to the same side or raises the pelvis toward the ribs on that side. Bilaterally, the QL extends the spine.

Low back exercises include one or more of the following muscles: Quadratus Lumborum, Erector Spinae, Multifidi, Intertranversarii.

Calisthenics – 12 exercises
Stability Balls – 12 exercises
Tubing – 7 exercises
Weights – 7 exercises
Machines – 7 exercises
Medicine Balls – 15 exercises

Upper Body Extension

With pillow supporting abdomen, clasp hands behind back and lift upper body from floor. Keep chin tucked while lifting.

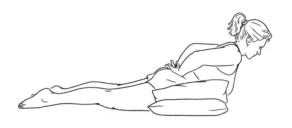

Hip Extension: Prone

Lift one leg from floor, keeping knee locked.

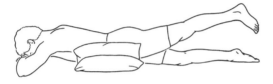

Arm / Leg Lift: Opposite: Prone

Lift one leg and opposite arm from floor, keeping knee locked.

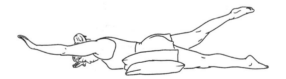

Hip Extension: All-Fours

Lift one leg backward with knee slightly flexed. Do not arch neck or back.

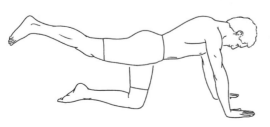

Upper Body Extension: All-Fours

Raise one arm in front. Do not arch
neck. Be sure to keep back flat.

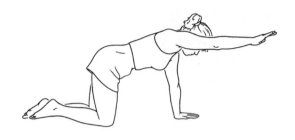

Arm / Leg Extension: Alternate All-Fours

Raise one arm and opposite
leg. Do not arch neck.

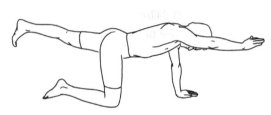

Hip Extension: Unilateral – Support

Torso on table, lift one leg, knee bent.

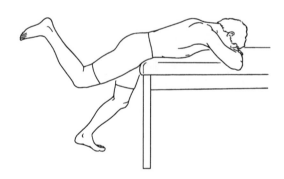

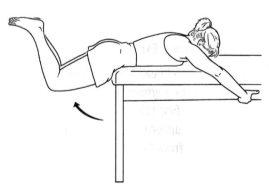

Hip Extension: Bilateral – Support

Torso on table, raise both legs, knees bent.

Extension: Prone

Lift upper body and legs from floor. Do not arch neck.

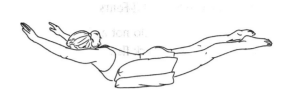

Lumbar Side Bend: Over Edge – Partner (Side-Lying)

On side, partner stabilizing pelvis and legs, raise trunk over edge of bed or table.

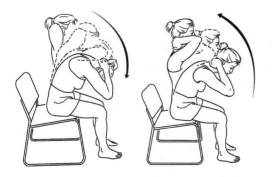

Lumbar Side Bend: Partner – Side-Lying

On side, partner stabilizing pelvis and legs, raise trunk.

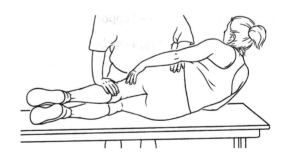

Segmental Flexion / Extension

Clasp hands behind head and slowly bend down, segment by segment, through lower back. To return, first raise chin, then straighten neck, upper back, and so on. Option: Extend from low back first.

Bridging: Double Leg (Gymball)

Lie on back, calves on ball. Slowly raise and lower buttocks.

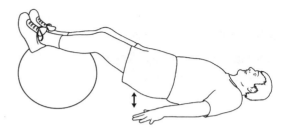

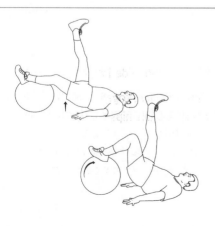

Bridging: Single Leg (Gymball)

Lie on back, calves on ball. With one leg vertical, slowly raise and lower buttocks.

Hamstring Curl: Double Leg (Gymball)

Lie on back, calves on ball, buttocks on floor. Raise buttocks then roll ball toward buttocks.

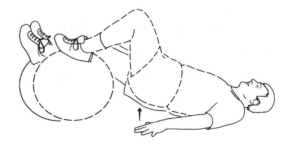

Hamstring Curl: Single Leg (Gymball)

Lie on back, calves on ball. Raise buttocks and hold. With one leg vertical, roll ball toward buttocks.

Extension: Prone (Dumbbell)

Hold dumbbell in front of chest
and extend low back.

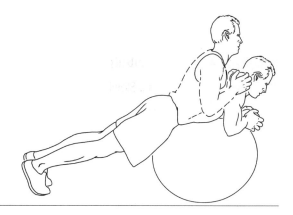

Hip Hinge: Double Leg (Gymball)

From sitting, roll out so ball supports shoulder
blades, back straight, knees over ankles.
Lower and raise hips, keeping back straight.

Hip Lift: Side Lying (Gymball)

Lie on side with feet together on ball. Support
head with hand. Lift hips in line with knees.

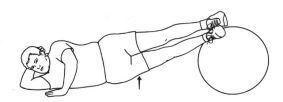

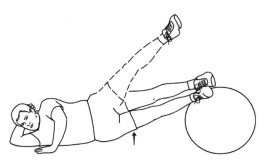

Hip Lift / Leg Lift: Side Lying (Gymball)

Lie on side with feet together on ball. Support
head with hand. Lift hips then lift top leg.

Arm Raise: Alternating – Prone

On hands and toes, over ball, raise arm and return. Repeat with other arm.

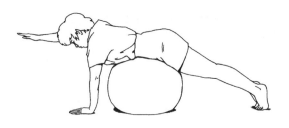

Leg Raise: Alternating – Prone

On hands and toes, over ball, raise one leg and return. Do not arch back. Repeat with other leg.

Arm and Leg Raise: Opposite – Prone

On hands and toes, over ball, raise one arm and opposite leg simultaneously. Do not arch back. Repeat with other limbs.

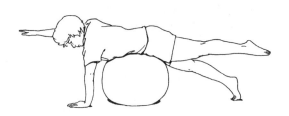

Arm and Leg Raise: Same-Side – Prone

On hands and toes, over ball, raise same-side arm and leg simultaneously. Do not arch back. Repeat with other side.

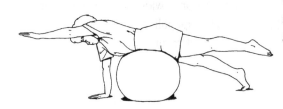

Scapular Retraction: Bilateral

Facing anchor, pull arms back, bringing shoulder blades together.

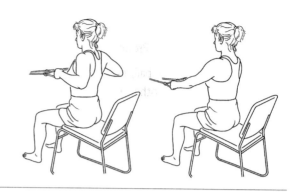

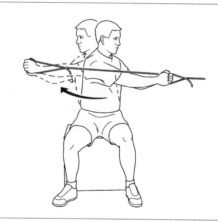

Lumbar Forward Rotation: Resisted – Sitting

With side toward anchor, gently rotate away from anchor in a pain-free range of motion.

Rotation: Resisted – Sitting

Sitting, side toward anchor, reach toward anchor, thumbs up, pull away from anchor. Keep arm furthest from anchor straight.

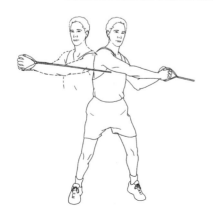

Rotation: Resisted – Standing

Side toward anchor in wide stance, reach toward anchor. Thumbs up, pull away from anchor. Keep arm furthest from anchor straight.

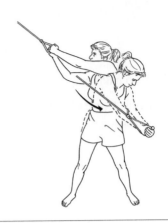

Lumbar Diagonal 1 Rotation: Resisted – Standing

With side toward anchor, reach up
and out toward anchor. Bend body,
rotating down to other side.

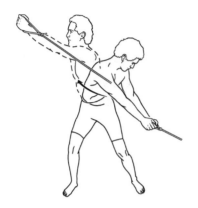

Lumbar Diagonal 2 Rotation: Resisted – Standing

With side toward anchor, feet slightly offset,
reach down across body toward anchor.
Straighten upper body, rotating up to other side.

Side Bend: Standing

Side toward anchor in wide stance, arms
above head, tilt trunk toward anchor. Grasp
handle and pull away from anchor.

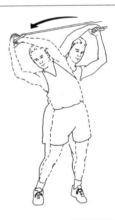

Dead Lift: Three Quarter (Barbell)

From three quarter squat position, straighten legs, keeping head up and back straight.

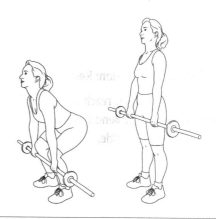

Dead Lift: Straight Leg (Barbell)

Bent 90° at hips, legs straight, back flat, raise torso until in line with legs.

Dead Lift (Barbell)

From squat, straighten legs, keeping head up and back straight.

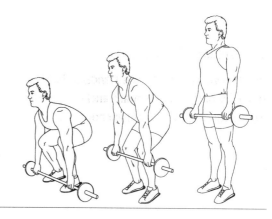

Good Morning (Barbell)

Bent 90° at hips, knees slightly bent, head up, back straight, raise torso until in line with legs.

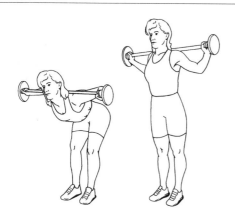

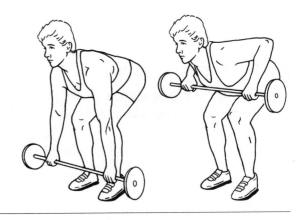

Row: Bent Over (Barbell)

Lift barbell to chest, keeping back flat and knees bent.

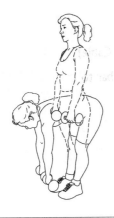

Dead Lift (Dumbbell)

Bent 90° at hips, legs straight, back flat, raise torso until in line with legs.

Dead Lift: Twisting (Dumbbell)

Legs straight, back flat, torso twisted, hold dumbbells at outside of one foot. Bring body up, twisting to forward. Alternate sides.

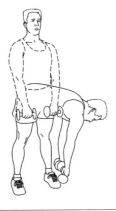

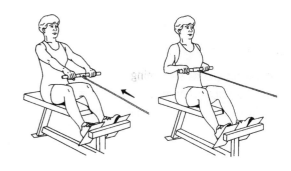

Row (Cable)

Torso erect, pull bar to lower chest.

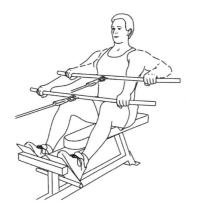

Row: Wide Grip (Cable)

Torso erect, pull bar to chest.

Row (V-Bar, Cable)

Torso erect, pull bar to chest.

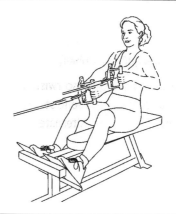

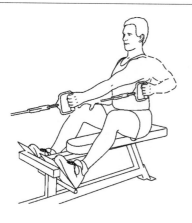

Row: Single Arm (Cable)

Torso erect, bracing other hand on thigh, pull arm back to side of chest.

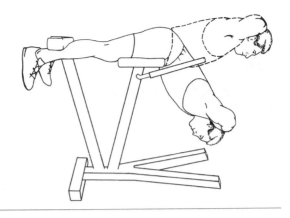

Extension

Bent at hips, back straight, hands behind head, raise torso until in line with legs. Do NOT extend past parallel to floor.

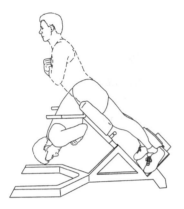

Extension: Incline

Bent at hips, back straight, hands crossed on chest, raise torso until in line with legs.

Extension (Machine)

Torso forward, back straight, extend torso backward, until it aligns with hips.

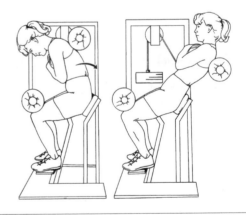

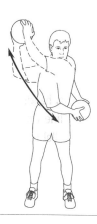

Trunk: Hip Chop

Hold medicine ball at one hip. Quickly move ball from hip to above opposite shoulder and quickly return.

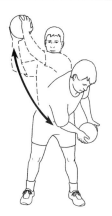

Trunk: Knee Chop

Hold medicine ball outside of knee. Quickly move ball from knee to above opposite shoulder and return quickly.

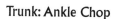

Trunk: Ankle Chop

Hold medicine ball outside of ankle. Quickly move ball from ankle to above opposite shoulder and return quickly.

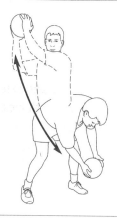

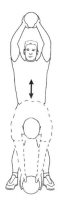

Trunk: Flexion / Extension (Standing)

Hold medicine ball over head. Touch ball to floor, bending knees as necessary.

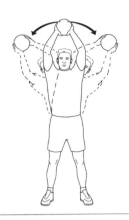

Trunk: Lateral Bend – Standing

Hold medicine ball over head. Bend
to one side, then the other.

Trunk: Flexion / Extension – Sitting

Sit holding a medicine ball between legs. Raise
ball over head. Return to starting position.

Trunk: Rotation

Stand with back to counter. Hold a ball.
Turn and place medicine ball on counter.
Twist to opposite side and pick up ball.
Turn and place ball on counter.

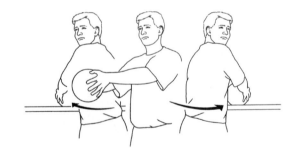

Trunk: Extension – Prone

Lie prone, holding medicine ball out in
front. Lift chest and ball off floor.

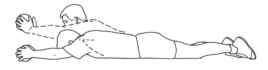

Trunk: Extension with Rotation – Prone

Lie prone, holding medicine ball out in front. Lift and rotate upper body to one side and then the other, ball off floor.

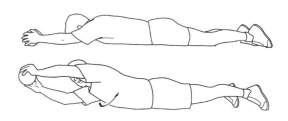

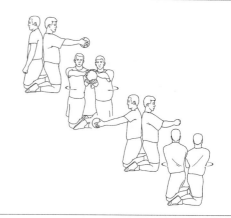

Partner Drill: Half Twist – Standing

Holding medicine ball, stand back-to-back. Turn to side and pass ball. Rotate to other side and receive ball.

Partner Drill: Half Twist – Kneeling

Holding medicine ball, kneel back-to-back. Turn to side and pass ball. Rotate to other side and receive ball.

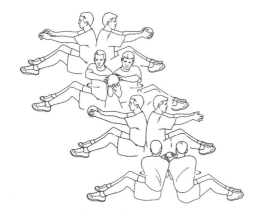

Partner Drill: Half Twist – Sitting

Holding medicine ball, sit back-to-back. Turn to side and pass ball. Rotate to other side and receive ball.

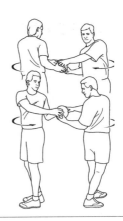

Partner Drill: Full Twist – Standing

Holding medicine ball, stand with back to partner, 1-2 feet apart. Rotate and pass ball behind. Rotate to other side and receive ball behind.

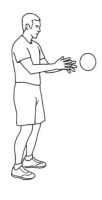

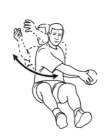

Partner Drill: Lateral Pass

Holding medicine ball at far hip, sit several feet from partner. Rotate and toss ball. Catch ball as it returns.

Partner Drill: Rotational Pass – Two-Handed

Holding medicine ball, stand several feet from partner. Rotate away and back, tossing ball. Partner catches ball and does same.

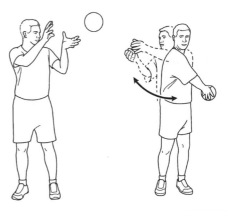

Chapter 9: Forearm Exercises

The muscles of the forearm are complex in their alignment and functions. They will be divided into five groups: flexors, extensors, supinators, pronators, and radial or ulnar flexors. The flexors are comprised of both the ulnar and radial flexors, which originate off the distal humerus. The extensors are comprised of the radial and ulnar extensors, and originate off the distal humerus. The supinators consist of the biceps brachii and the supinator. The pronators are two small muscles, proximally the pronator teres, distally the pronator quadratus. The radial flexors are the brachioradialis, radial flexors, and radial extensors working in concert to bend the thumb side of the hand toward the forearm. The ulnar flexors are the ulnar flexor and extensor working together to bend the wrist toward the ulna.

Forearm exercises include one or more of the following muscles: Radial Flexors, Ulnar Flexors, Pronator Teres, Pronator Quadratus, Supinator, and Biceps Brachii.

> Flexion – 12 exercises
> Extension – 6 exercises
> Rotation – 4 exercises
> Lateral / Medial Deviation – 4 exercises

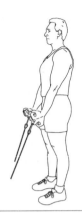

Wrist Curl: Standing (Cable)

Knees slightly bent, flex wrists up as far
as possible, keeping arms straight.

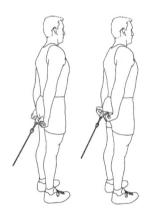

Wrist Curl: Behind Back – Standing (Cable)

Knees slightly bent, flex wrists up as far
as possible, keeping arms straight.

Wrist Curl: Behind Back – Standing (Barbell)

Knees slightly bent, flex wrists up as far
as possible, keeping arms straight.

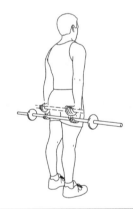

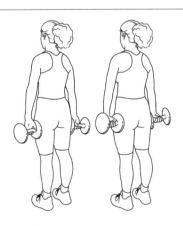

Wrist Curl: Behind Back – Standing (Dumbbell)

Knees slightly bent, flex wrists up as far
as possible, keeping arms straight.

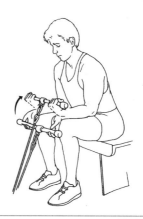

Wrist Curl: Sitting (Cable)

Flex wrists up toward body, keeping forearms on thighs.

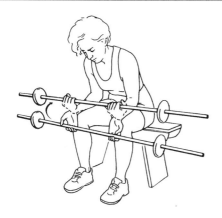

Wrist Curl: Sitting (Barbell)

Flex wrists up toward body. Keep forearms on thighs.

Wrist Curl: Sitting (Dumbbell)

Flex wrists up toward body, keeping forearms on thighs.

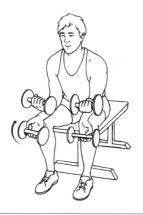

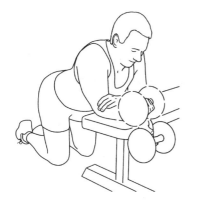

Wrist Curl: Single Arm – Kneeling (Dumbbell)

Holding forearm stationary with other hand, flex wrist up as far as possible.

Wrist Curl: Kneeling (Barbell)

Flex wrists up as far as possible, keeping forearms in contact with bench.

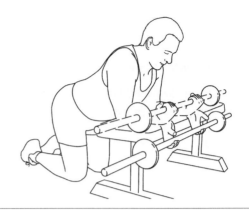

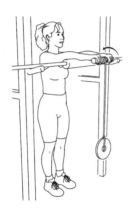

Wrist Curl: Reverse Grip – Standing (Wrist Roller)

Arms straight, support between elbow and wrist. Using reverse grip, roll rope onto bar by extending wrists back, alternating hands.

Wrist Flexion: Resisted

With tubing wrapped around left fist and other end secured under foot, bend wrist up (palm up) as far as possible. Keep forearm on thigh.

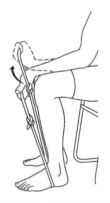

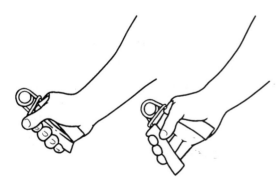

Hand Gripper

Squeeze grip as tightly as possible, then release.

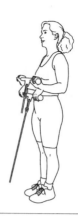

Wrist Curl: Reverse Grip – Standing (Cable)

Knees slightly bent, using reverse grip, elbows bent to 90°, extend wrists back as far as possible.

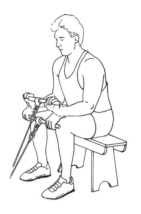

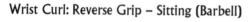

Wrist Curl: Reverse Grip – Sitting (Cable)

Using reverse grip, extend wrists back toward body. Keep forearms on thighs.

Wrist Curl: Reverse Grip – Sitting (Barbell)

Using reverse grip, extend wrists back toward body. Keep forearms on thighs.

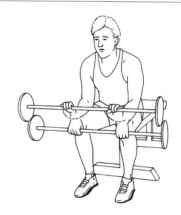

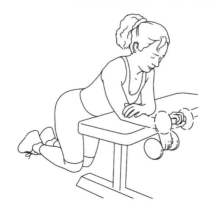

Wrist Curl: Single Arm, Reverse Grip – Kneeling (Dumbbell)

Hold forearm stationary with other hand. Using reverse grip, extend wrist back as far as possible.

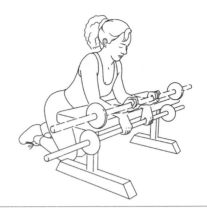

Wrist Curl: Reverse Grip – Kneeling (Barbell)

Using reverse grip, extend wrists back as far as possible. Keep forearms in contact with bench.

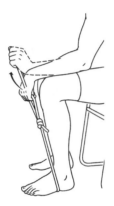

Wrist Extension: Resisted

With tubing wrapped around left fist and other end secured under foot, bend wrist up (palm down) as far as possible. Keep forearm on thigh.

Rotation: Single Arm (Dumbbell)

Holding forearm with other hand, slowly rotate hand as far as possible to one side, then the other.

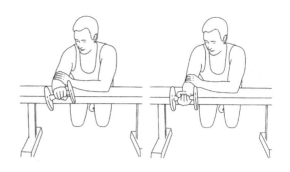

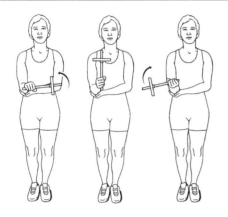

Rotation: Single Arm (Thor's Hammer)

Holding forearm with other hand, slowly rotate hand to one side then the other, as far as possible.

Forearm Supination: Resisted

With palm down, stabilize forearm on thigh with other hand. Keep tubing to inside of hand and roll palm up as far as possible.

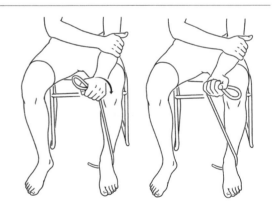

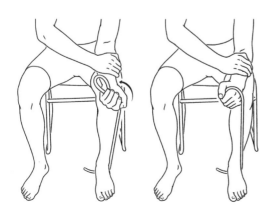

Forearm Pronation: Resisted

With palm up, stabilize forearm on thigh with other hand. Keep tubing to outside of hand and roll palm down as far as possible.

Wrist Radial Deviation: Resisted – Standing

With arm at side, thumb forward, a weight in hand, bend wrist back. Return {slowly, rapidly, moderately}.

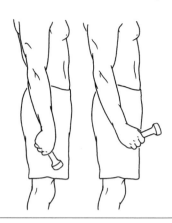

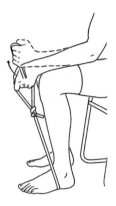

Radial Deviation: Resisted

With tubing wrapped around fist and other end secured under foot, bend wrist up (thumb side up) as far as possible. Keep forearm on thigh.

Wrist Ulnar Deviation: Resisted – Standing

With arm at side, thumb forward, a weight in hand, bend wrist forward. Return {slowly, rapidly, moderately}.

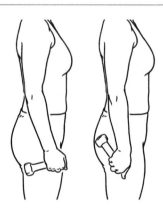

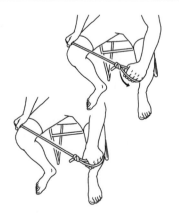

Ulnar Deviation: Resisted

With tubing wrapped around fist and other end secured, palm down, bend wrist out to side (thumb in) as far as possible. Keep forearm braced on knee.

Chapter 10: Rotator Cuff Exercises

The infamous rotator cuff is a group of four small muscles that provides joint support for the shoulder (glenohumeral) joint. These muscles generally work eccentrically to maintain the humeral head in the center of the socket of the scapula. The role of the rotator cuff is indispensable for proper shoulder mechanics and if injured or atrophied, the shoulder will operate improperly, even though other muscles will try to compensate. It will also hurt to move the arm off the side of the body in abduction. There are many syndromes in which the cuff is involved, but with proper training, one can prevent many of the traditional resistance and sports training injuries.

The rotator cuff consists of three external rotators: infraspinatus, supraspinatus, and teres minor, and one internal rotator: the subscapularis. Exercises for these muscles will rotate the humerus along its lengthwise axis. These muscles are tonic or postural not phasic and therefore are not the kind that will hypertrophy. Thus, most training for them is for endurance and function, not with high loads or for power, although some rehabilitation and pre-habilitation exercises will progress to plyometrics in preparation for sports movements.

Rotator Cuff exercises include one or more of the following muscles: Subscapularis, Supraspinatus, Infraspinatus, Teres Minor, Biceps Brachii, Lower and Middle Trapezius, and Rhomboids.

Internal Rotation – 16 exercises
External Rotation – 18 exercises
Diagonal – 5 exercises
Scaption – 3 exercises
Periscapulars – 6 exercises
Stabilization / Proprioception – 10 exercises

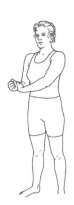

Internal Rotation: Isometric

Keeping elbow at side, use other hand at wrist to apply {light, moderate, maximal} resistance to inward motion. Hold.

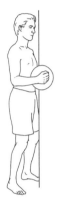

Internal Rotation: Isometric

Using door frame for resistance, press palm of one hand into ball using {light, moderate, maximal} pressure. Keep elbow in at side. Hold.

Horizontal Adduction: Isometric

Using door frame for resistance, press inner arm into ball using {light, moderate, maximal} pressure. Keep upper arm parallel to floor, elbow bent 90°. Hold.

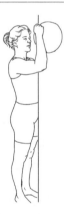

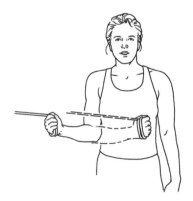

Internal Rotation – Active Resisted

Hold tubing in one hand, elbow at side and forearm out. Rotate forearm in across body.

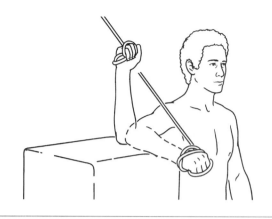

Internal Rotation in 90° of Abduction

Anchor behind, tubing around one hand, elbow bent 90°, forearm up, pull forearm forward, keeping elbow bent.

Internal Rotation in Abduction – Single Arm

Face away from anchor in shoulder width stance. Bend elbow to 90°, forearm up, arm out to side. Palm forward, pull forearm down, keeping elbow bent.

Internal Rotation in Flexion – Single Arm

Side toward anchor in shoulder width stance, bend elbow to 90°, forearm up, arm in front. Palm in, pull forearm down, keeping elbow bent.

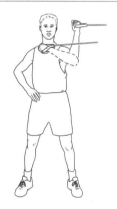

Internal Rotation: Progressive Resisted – Side-Lying

Holding weight, raise forearm toward body, keeping elbow at side.

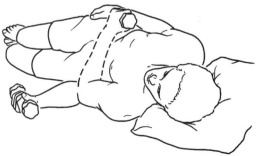

Internal Rotation: Side-Lying (Dumbbell)

Elbow steady, rotate forearm toward trunk.

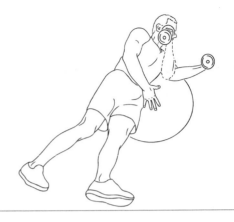

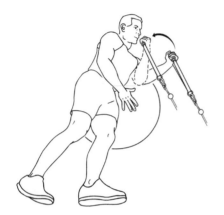

Internal Rotation: Side-Lying (Cable)

Elbow steady, rotate forearm toward trunk.

Upper Extremity: 90/90 Throw – Half-Kneeling

Holding medicine ball in one hand, kneel on same side knee. Throw ball forward to partner. Catch ball as it returns.

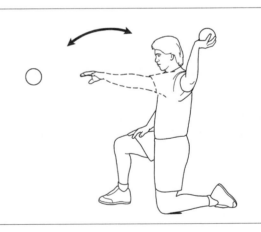

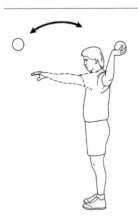

Upper Extremity: 90/90 Throw – Standing

In shoulder width stance, hold medicine ball, in one hand. Throw ball forward to partner. Catch ball as it returns.

Upper Extremity: 90/90 Throw – Split Stance

Stand with foot forward on non-throwing side. Hold medicine ball, in left hand. Throw ball forward to partner. Catch ball as it returns.

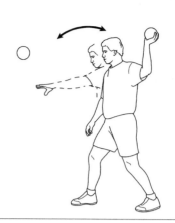

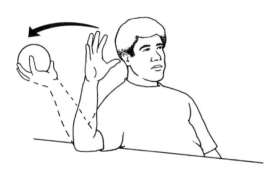

Upper Extremity: Catch / Stretch

Sit at table with arm supported. Catch medicine ball thrown by partner.

Upper Extremity: Catch / Stretch / Throw

Sit at table with arm supported. Catch medicine ball and throw back to partner.

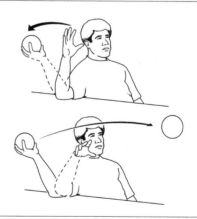

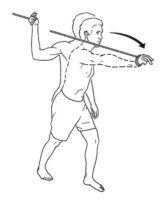

Functional Pattern Strengthening: Serving / Throwing

Hold tubing behind, with one hand. Pull forward as though serving in tennis or throwing a ball.

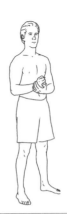

External Rotation: Isometric

Keeping elbow at side, use other hand at wrist to apply {light, moderate, maximal} resistance to outward motion.

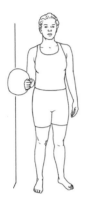

External Rotation: Isometric

Using wall to provide resistance, and keeping right arm at side, press back of hand into ball using {light, moderate, maximal} pressure.

Isometric Horizontal Abduction: Isometric

Using wall for resistance, press outside of arm into ball using {light, moderate, maximal} pressure. Keep upper arm parallel to floor, elbow bent 90°.

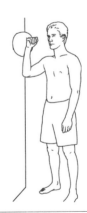

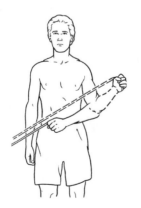

External Rotation: Active Resisted

Hold tubing in one hand, elbow at side and forearm across body. Rotate forearm out.

External Rotation in 90° of Abduction

Facing anchor, tubing around hand, elbow bent 90°, forearm forward, pull forearm back, keeping elbow bent.

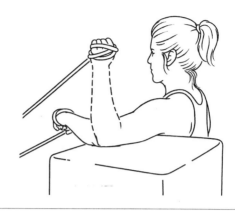

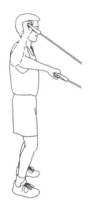

External Rotation in Abduction – Single Arm

Face anchor in shoulder width stance with elbow bent at 90°, forearm in front. Palm down, pull forearm up.

External Rotation in Flexion – Single Arm

Side toward anchor in shoulder width stance with elbow bent at 90°, arm across body. Palm down, pull forearm up, keeping elbow bent.

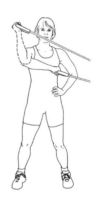

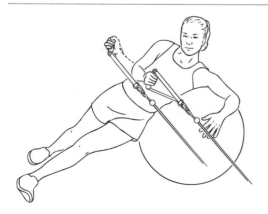

External Rotation: Single Side-Lying (Cable)

Elbow steady, rotate forearm out. Repeat with other arm.

External Rotation: Prone

Lie with left upper arm straight out from body, elbow bent to 90°, weight in hand. Rotate forearm up, keeping elbow bent. Return slowly, rapidly, moderately.

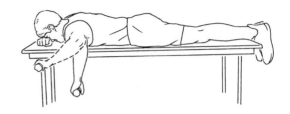

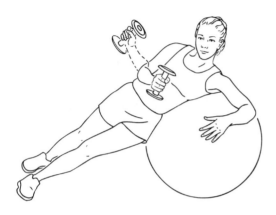

External Rotation: Single – Side-Lying (Dumbbell)

Elbow steady, rotate forearm out.
Repeat with other arm.

Resisted External Rotation: Abduction – Bilateral

Face anchor, tubing end in each hand. Keep arms elevated and elbows bent to 90°, forearms forward. Pinch shoulder blades together and rotate forearms up.

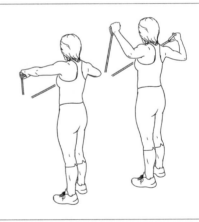

External Rotation: Prone

Back straight, shoulders and elbows at 90°, raise forearms to horizontal.

External Rotation: Progressive Resisted – (Side-Lying)

Holding weight, towel under arm, raise right forearm toward ceiling. Keep elbow bent and at side.

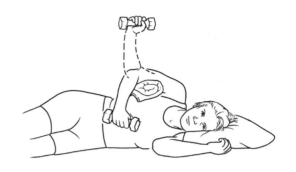

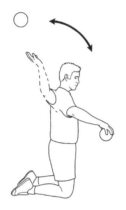

Upper Extremity: 90/90 Reverse Throw – Kneeling

Kneel, holding medicine ball in one hand. Throw ball backward over shoulder to a partner. Catch ball as it returns.

Upper Extremity: 90/90 Reverse Throw – Half-Kneeling

Holding medicine ball in one hand, kneel on same side knee. Throw ball backward over shoulder to partner. Catch ball as it returns.

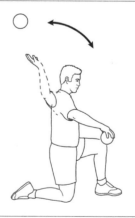

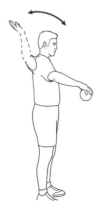

Upper Extremity: 90/90 Reverse Throw – Standing

In shoulder width stance, hold medicine ball in one hand. Throw ball backward over shoulder to partner. Catch ball as it returns.

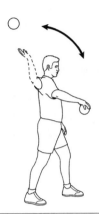

Upper Extremity: 90/90 Reverse Throw – Split Stance

Stand with foot forward on non-throwing side. Hold medicine ball in one hand. Throw ball backward over shoulder to a partner. Catch ball as it returns.

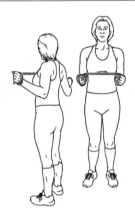

External Rotation: Resisted, in Neutral – Bilateral

Sit or stand, tubing in both hands, elbows at sides, bent to 90°, forearms forward. Pinch shoulder blades together and rotate forearms out. Keep elbows at sides.

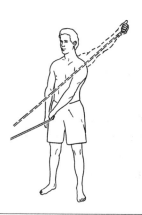

Diagonal: Resisted

Hold tubing with arm down across body, thumb pointing back. Pull arm up and out, rotating arm to palm forward.

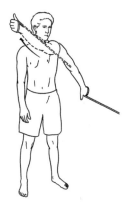

Diagonal: Resisted

Hold tubing with arm down and out from side, thumb down. Pull arm across body and over head, rotating arm to thumb up.

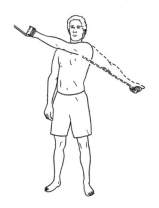

Diagonal Extension: Resisted

Hold tubing with arm across body above shoulder, palm down. Gently pull down and away from body, rotating arm to palm up.

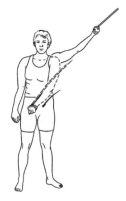

Diagonal Extension: Resisted

Hold tubing with arm above and behind, palm up. Bring arm down across body, rotating to palm down.

Trunk: Hip Chop

Hold a medicine ball at one hip. Quickly
move ball from hip to above opposite
shoulder and quickly return.

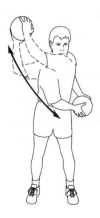

Scaption with External Rotation

Holding weight, raise arm diagonally from hip to above head. Keep elbow straight, thumb up.

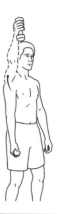

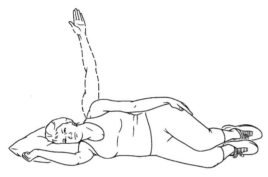

Abduction: Side-Lying

Lie on one side. Raise arm above head. Keep palm forward.

Supraspinatus Strengthening

Holding weight, raise arm diagonally from hip to just below shoulder level. Keep elbow straight, thumb down.

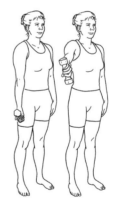

Horizontal Abduction with External Rotation – Prone

Holding weights, raise arms out from sides, pinching shoulder blades. Keep elbows straight, thumbs up.

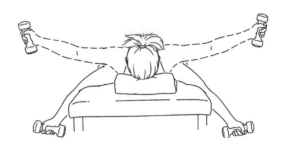

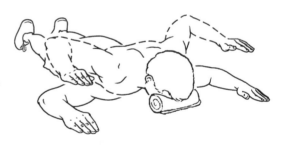

Horizontal Abduction with Interior Rotation – Prone

Holding weights, raise arms out from sides, pinching shoulder blades. Keep elbows straight, thumbs down.

Scapular Retraction: Abduction – Prone

Lie with upper arms straight out from sides, elbows bent to 90°. Pinch shoulder blades together and raise arms a few inches from floor.

Scapular: Flexion – Prone

Holding weights, raise both arms forward. Keep elbows straight.

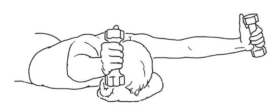

Extension: Progressive Resisted – Prone

Holding weights, arms back, raise arms from floor, keeping elbows straight.

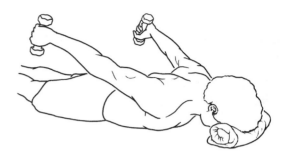

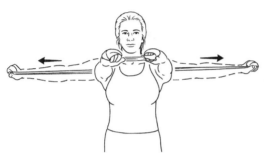

Chest Pull – Resisted

With resistive band looped around each hand, and arms straight out in front, stretch band across chest.

Gymball on Wall: Clockwise / Counterclockwise

Stand away from wall with one hand supporting a ball on the wall. Lean into ball and move ball in circles clockwise.

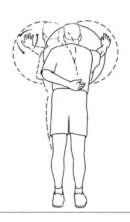

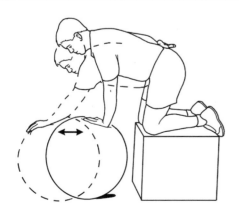

Gymball on Wall: Partner Resistance

Stand away from wall. Support ball with one hand. Resist as partner attempts to push your arm up. Don't let your arm move.

Hand on Ball: Side to Side

Kneel on surface level with top of ball. Place one hand on ball. Maintain shoulders over ball. Move ball side to side.

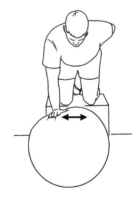

Hand on Ball: Front to Back

Kneel on surface level with top of ball. Place one hand on ball. Maintain shoulders over ball. Move ball forward to back.

Hand on Ball: Diagonal

Kneel on surface level with top of ball. Place one hand on ball. Maintain shoulders over ball. Move ball in diagonal pattern, forward to back, alternating directions.

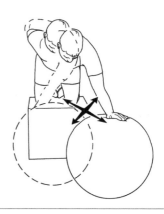

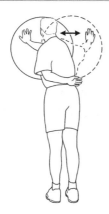

Hand on Ball: Circle – Clockwise / Counterclockwise

Kneel on surface level with top of ball. Place one hand on ball. Maintain shoulders over ball. Move ball in circles clockwise.

Hand on Ball: Partner Resist

Kneel on surface, level with top of ball. Place one hand on ball. Maintain shoulders over ball. Resist arm movement as partner attempts to push you {forward, backward, side to side, in circle} at {arm, shoulder, trunk}.

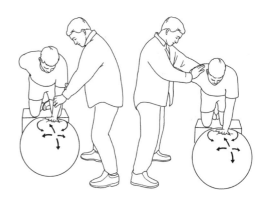

Gymball on Wall: Side to Side

Stand away from wall with one hand supporting a ball on the wall. Lean into ball and move ball side to side.

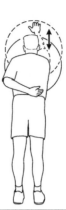

Gymball on Wall: Up and Down

Stand away from wall with one hand supporting a ball on the wall. Lean into ball and move ball up and down.

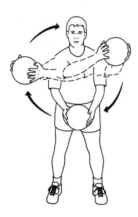

Trunk: Circle

Hold medicine ball with arms straight. Rapidly move arms in circle counterclockwise.

Chapter 11: Neck Exercises

The neck is comprised of seven cervical vertebrae and their linkage to the skull. It moves in three planes: flexion / extension, lateral bending, and rotation — separately or in combination. With its role in encasing the spinal cord, and its large and many ranges of motion, the neck is extremely vulnerable to certain kinds of injury that can impact both the quality of life and life itself. Therefore, strengthening the neck, especially for athletics, is a worthwhile goal.

Conditioning through the full ranges of motion is appropriate although, as we age, it is recommended we not go to the extremes of neck extension. As postural muscles, except for the trapezius itself, neck training is done either isometrically or with very light loads and high repetitions.

Neck exercises include one or more of the following muscles: Trapezius, Levator Scapula, Sternocleidomastoid, Scalenes, and Intervertebral Muscles (not shown).

    Extension – 9 exercises
    Flexion – 9 exercises
    Rotation – 3 exercises
    Lateral Flexion – 9 exercises

Extension: Isometric (in Neutral)

Using light pressure from fingertips at back of head, resist bending head backward.

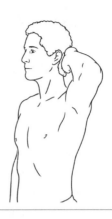

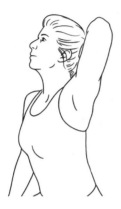

Extension: Isometric (Out of Neutral)

Bend head backward. Apply Light pressure to back of head with fingertips and resist bending head further backward.

Extension: Lying – Resist (Hand)

Hand applying resistance on back of head, move head toward back.

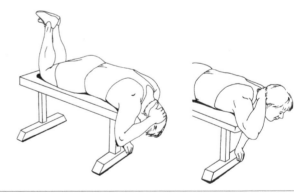

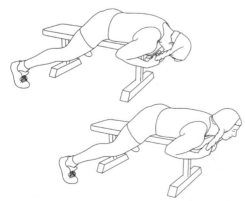

Lying – Resist (Towel)

Place towel on head and roll ends to hold in place. Move head toward back, applying resistance with towel.

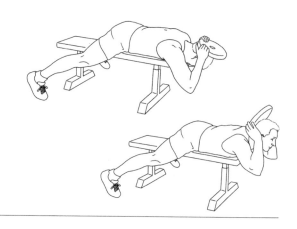

Extension: Lying – Resist (Plate)

Holding light weight against back of head, move head toward back.

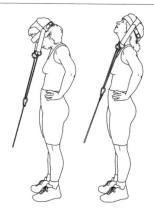

Extension: Standing (Cable Head Harness)

Move head toward back.

Extension: Sitting (Cable Head Harness)

Hands on knees for support, move head toward back.

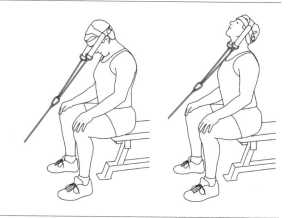

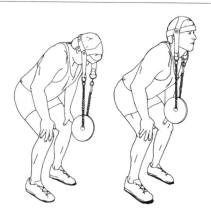

Extension: Standing (Head Harness)

Hands on knees for support, move head toward back.

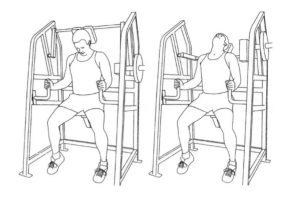

Extension (Machine)

Back of head on pad, move head toward back.

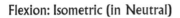

Flexion: Isometric (in Neutral)

Using light pressure from fingertips at forehead, resist bending head forward.

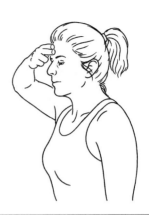

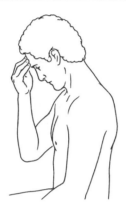

Flexion: Isometric (Out of Neutral)

Bend head forward. Apply light pressure to forehead with fingertips and resist bending head further forward.

Flexion: Lying – Resist (Hand)

Hand applying resistance on forehead, move head toward chest.

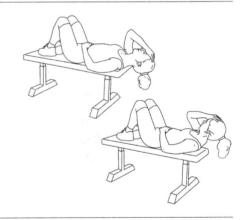

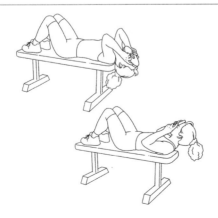

Flexion: Lying – Resist (Plate)

Holding light weight against forehead, move head toward chest.

Flexion: Lying (Head Harness)

Holding head harness, move head toward chest.

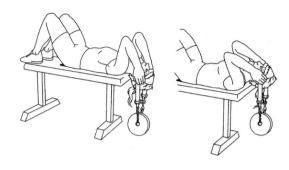

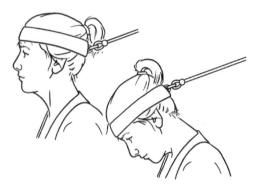

Flexion: Resisted – Inner Range

Stand or sit with high anchor behind, band at back of head strap. From upright, bend head toward chest.

Flexion: Standing (Cable Head Harness)

Move head toward chest.

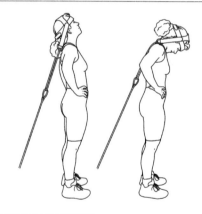

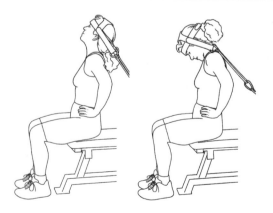

Flexion: Sitting (Cable Head Harness)

Move head toward chest.

Flexion (Machine)

Face and forehead on pad, move head toward chest.

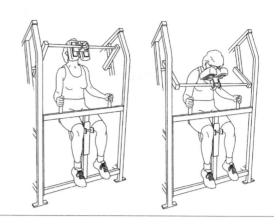

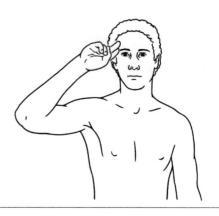

Rotation: Isometric (in Neutral)

Using light pressure from fingertips at
right temple, resist turning head.

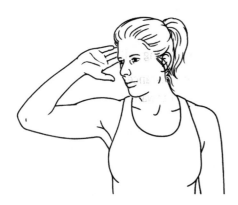

Rotation: Isometric (Out of Neutral)

Turn head to right side. Apply light pressure
to temple and resist turning head further.
Turn head to other side and repeat.

Rotation: Resisted – Inner Range

Stand or sit with left side toward head
height anchor, band at back of head
strap. Turn head toward anchor.

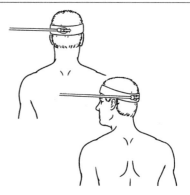

Lateral Bend – Isometric (in Neutral)

Using light pressure from fingertips, press into right temple. Resist bending head sideways.

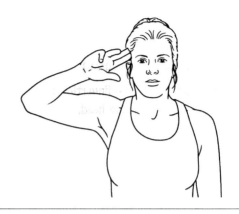

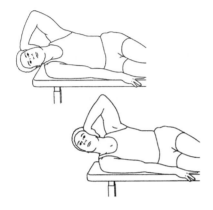

Flexion: Lateral, Lying – Resist (Hand)

Hand applying resistance on side of head, move head toward shoulder.

Flexion: Lateral (Machine)

Side of head against pad, move head toward shoulder.

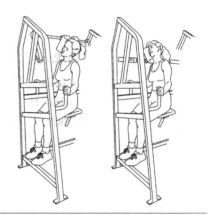

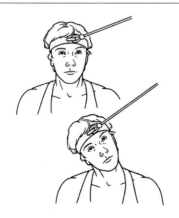

Side Bend: Resisted – Inner Range

Stand or sit with left side toward high anchor, band at front of head strap. Bend ear toward shoulder, away from anchor.

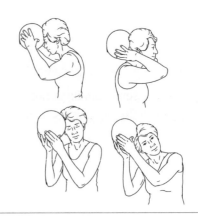

Beach Ball Strengthening: Isometric

Sitting or standing, hold ball against wall. Press head gently into ball in each of the positions shown.

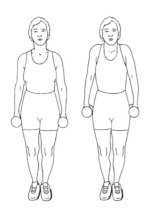

Shrug (Dumbbell)

Knees slightly bent, raise shoulders as high as possible, keeping arms straight.

Shrug: Medium Grip (Barbell)

Knees slightly bent, raise shoulders as high as possible, keeping arms straight.

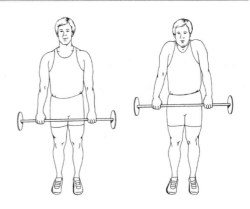

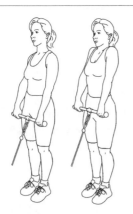

Shrug (Cable)

Knees slightly bent, raise shoulders as high as possible keeping arms straight.

Shrug: Wide Grip (Machine)

Knees slightly bent, raise shoulders as
high as possible, keeping arms straight.

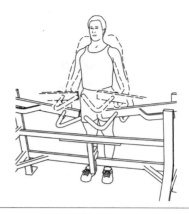

Chapter 12: Finger / Hand Exercises

The hand and finger muscles are many and complex, especially around the thumb. For simplicity sake, the movements can be divided into two main groups — fingers and thumb — with each having its own ranges of motion. The fingers can flex/extend, abduct/adduct, and circumduct (a combination of all four movements). Contraction of the flexors and/or extensors on the medial side of one finger and the lateral side of an adjacent finger allows for adduction/abduction movements. The thumb, while technically a saddle-joint, operates like a ball-and-socket joint with the same single plane movements of the fingers plus rotation. Exercises that require forearm flexion or extension factor into hand and finger exercises. Forearm rotations do not play into hand and finger movements.

Finger/Hand muscles include too many small muscles to list; they can be divided into: Finger Flexors, Finger Extensors, Finger Abductors, and Thumb muscles.

Finger / Hand – 12 exercises

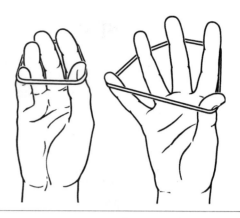

Finger Extension / Thumb Abduction: Resisted

With rubber band around one thumb and all fingers, hand slightly cupped, gently spread thumb and fingers apart.

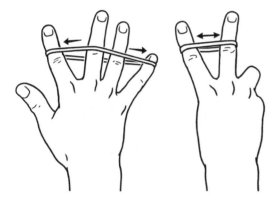

Finger Abduction: Resisted

With rubber band around two or more fingers of one hand, gently spread fingers apart.

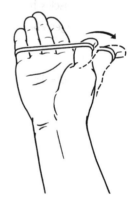

Thumb Extension: Resisted

With palm up, with rubber band around fingers and thumb, move thumb outward.

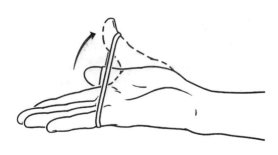

Thumb Abduction: Resisted

With palm up, with rubber band around fingers and thumb, move thumb up away from palm.

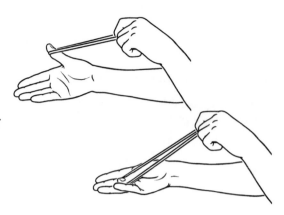

Thumb Opposition: Resisted

With rubber band around thumb, hold other end with other hand. Rotate thumb up and over toward little finger. Repeat toward each finger.

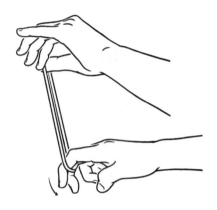

Finger Flexion: Resisted

With rubber band around two or more fingers of one hand, hold other end with other hand. Curl fingers toward palm.

Thumb Flexion: Resisted

With rubber band around thumb, hold other end with other hand. Bend thumb toward palm.

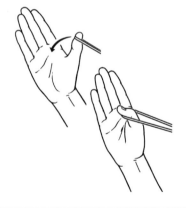

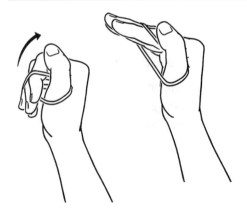

Finger Extension: Resisted

With one hand in fist, wrap rubber band around thumb and back of fingers. Keeping first row of knuckles bent, slowly straighten fingers.

Finger Flexion: Resisted

Apply {light, medium, heavy} resistance with other hand while curling fingers of one hand.

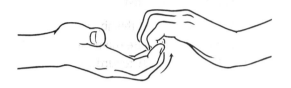

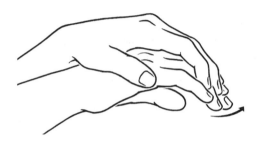

Finger Extension: Resisted

Apply {light, medium, heavy} resistance with other hand while extending fingers from middle knuckles of one hand.

Hand Gripper

Squeeze grip as tightly as possible, then release.

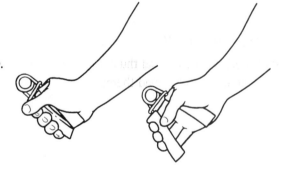

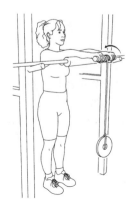

Wrist Curl: Reverse Grip – (Wrist Roller)

Arms straight, support between elbow and wrist. Using reverse grip, roll rope onto bar by extending wrists back, alternating hands.

About VHI

Visual Health Information (VHI) is the leading publisher of reproducible exercise tools. VHI has been producing exercise collections for the rehabilitation and fitness markets since 1980.

VHI produces reproducible exercise cards and computer software. VHI has over 35 different exercise collections. These collections include exercises for Outpatient Physical Therapy, Geriatrics, Pediatrics, Fitness, Strength & Conditioning, Pre/Postnatal, Speech, Pulmonary Rehab and much more.

The content for the Exercise Idea book series is derived from the over 9,000 exercise images in the VHI exercise database. These books are designed to show you the wide range of exercises that can be used for specific purposes.

To view all the VHI offerings and collections, visit **www.vhikits.com**, or call **1-800-356-0709.**